Social Work with Groups: Expanding Horizons

The *Social Work with Groups* series:

- *Group Work Reaching Out: People, Places and Power,* edited by James A. Garland

- *Social Work with Groups: Expanding Horizons,* edited by Stanley Wenocur, Paul H. Ephross, Thomas V. Vassil, and Raju K. Varghese

For information on previous issues of the *Social Work with Groups* series, edited by Catherine P. Papell and Beulah Rothman, please contact: The Haworth Press, Inc., 10 Alice Street, Binghamton, NY 13904-1580 USA.

Social Work with Groups: Expanding Horizons

Stanley Wenocur, PhD
Paul H. Ephross, PhD
Thomas V. Vassil, PhD
Raju K. Varghese, EdD, MPH
Editors

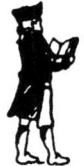

The Haworth Press, Inc.
New York • London • Norwood (Australia)

Social Work with Groups: Expanding Horizons has also been published as *Social Work with Groups*, Volume 16, Numbers 1/2 1993.

The Haworth Press, Inc., 10 Alice Street, Binghamton, NY 13904-1580 USA

Library of Congress Cataloging-in-Publication Data

Social work with groups : expanding horizons / Stanley Wenocur . . . [et al.], editors.
     p. cm.
    Published also as v. 16, no. 1/2 of the journal Social work with groups.
    Includes bibliographical references.
    ISBN 1-56024-296-5 (hard)
    1. Social group work–United States–Congresses. I. Wenocur, Stanley, 1938-.
HV45.S64 1993
361.4–dc20   92-34708
                                                               CIP

PLANNING COMMITTEE
FOR THE TENTH ANNUAL SYMPOSIUM
OF THE ASSOCIATION FOR THE ADVANCEMENT
OF SOCIAL WORK WITH GROUPS

Baltimore, Maryland
October 27-30, 1988

Paul H. Ephross and Thomas V. Vassil, co-chairs

Donald J. Carroll	*Sharon England*
Geoffrey Greif (abstracts)*	*Judith Haran*
Curtis Janzen (registration)*	*Harold Lipton*
Daniel Merlin (abstracts)*	*Margo Okazawa-Ray*
Ogden Rogers	*Kim Turner (social events)**
Raju K. Varghese (arrangements)*	*Joan C. Weiss*
Stanley Wenocur (publications)*	

* sub-committee chairs

BOARD OF DIRECTORS–AASWG–1988-89

Judith A.B. Lee, W. Hartford, CT, *President*
Ruby B. Pernell, Cleveland, OH, *Vice-President*
Marcos Leiderman, New Brunswick, NJ, *Secretary*
John H. Ramey, Akron, OH, *Membership Secretary*
Martin L. Birnbaum, New York, NY, *Treasurer*
Kenneth L. Chau, Long Beach, CA
Lise Darveau-Fournie, Montreal, P.Q.
Paul H. Ephross, Baltimore, MD
James E. Garland, Boston, MA
Charles Garvin, Ann Arbor, MI
Estelle Hopmeyer, Montreal, P.Q.
Alice Home, Montreal, P.Q.
Norma C. Lang, Toronto, Ont.
Catherine P. Papell, Garden City, NY
Beulah G. Rothman, Miami, FL
Thomas V. Vassil, Baltimore, MD
Elizabeth Lewis, Cleveland, OH

Social Work with Groups:
Expanding Horizons

CONTENTS

SELECTED PAPERS

ABOUT THE EDITORS

Stanley Wenocur, PhD, has a special interest in social change oriented work, work with task-oriented groups such as those involved in community action and management. He is the co-author of *From Charity to Enterprise* (University of Illinois Press, 1989), and is Associate Professor at the School of Social Community Planning, University of Maryland.

Paul Ephross, PhD, is a task oriented group worker, nationally known for his counseling and work with groups. He is Professor in the School of Social and Community Planning, University of Maryland.

Thomas Vassil, PhD, is Associate Professor at the School of Social and Community Planning, University of Maryland. His area of expertise is adolescents and he has done work with gangs. He and Paul Ephross are the co-authors of *Groups That Work* (Columbia University Press, 1988).

Raju Varghese, EdD, MPH, has a clinical background and is a certified social worker. He is interested in organization development. Currently, Associate Professor in the School of Social Work at the University of Maryland, he also has an appointment with the School of Medicine.

Introduction

For those who planned it, as well as for many of those who participated in it, the Tenth Annual Symposium on Social Work with Groups was an affirming experience. The Planning Committee, which I had the pleasure of co-chairing with Thomas Vassil, was itself an object lesson in group productivity in, as Mills phrases it, "the pursuit of a collective goal." The Symposium itself, both in its content and in the interaction it fostered among participants, illustrated the intimate interrelationships between process and product which are so central to group work theory and practice. The Committee's concern with the physical environment of the Symposium, its use of time, and its sequencing all resulted in affirming time-honored principles of group work.

Two aspects of the Symposium deserve special attention. The fact that this was the Tenth Annual Symposium provides an opportunity for a bit of reflection on past, present and future symposia. From this point of view, what was most striking about the Tenth Symposium was its combination of continuity and of change. Virtually all of the group work topics of the past several decades were represented, both overtly and implicitly, in the subject matter of the many presentations at the Symposium in Baltimore. Many sessions were concerned with the evolution of practice theory in group work. Many others were devoted to detailing the application and evolution of traditional group work techniques to new populations in need and to emerging needs of particular segments of the population. There was virtually unanimous recognition by Symposium participants of the supple and flexible characteristics of group work as a field, a method and a process.

This last point remains my most vivid memory of the Symposium's content and overall atmosphere. Rereading the group work classics of the period from 1930 to 1972, one is struck by their applicability, by their soundness, by the depth of their insights into the nature of the human condition, the interfacings between individuals, families, communities and broad societal processes and forms,

1

and most of all by their intense and unvarying humanity. The soundness and intellectual honesty of basic principles of group work theory and practice will, I trust, be as apparent at the hundredth symposium as they were at the tenth. So will the concern with social justice and its expression in the workings of organizations, communities and the specifics which affect live human beings.

The Tenth Annual Symposium provided the Committee and the Association for the Advancement of Social Work with Groups an opportunity to honor four of our colleagues. To our great pleasure, Dr. Ivor Echols, Professor and former Associate Dean of the School of Social Work of the University of Connecticut, and Abe Vinik, retired General Director of the Jewish Community Centers of Chicago, were able to participate in the Symposium and share reflections and observations with us which did much to enrich the Symposium. To our regret, the other two honorees could not participate in person: Robert Bond, retired Executive Director of the Cleveland Federation of Settlements was ill at the time of the Symposium, and Ray Richardson, former Executive Director of the Neighborhood House of Milwaukee, was honored posthumously.

The Tenth Symposium was the product of the generous investment of self on the part of too many people for all to be thanked individually. Particular thanks are due, however, to all of the members of the Planning Committee, whose names and special responsibilities are listed at the beginning of this volume, and to the volunteers who helped to staff the registration table and to perform the many other tasks which are relatively invisible but crucial to a successful symposium. To the Symposium co-chair, Thomas Vassil, and to my co-editors Raju Varghese and Stanley Wenocur, the field owes thanks for this publication. Stan Wenocur chaired the editorial committee and set an all-time record for the speed as well as the care with which manuscripts were prepared. The then new Dean of the School of Social Work at the University of Maryland at Baltimore, Dr. Ralph Dolgoff, contributed warm greetings and a warm reception and party to the Symposium. We express our gratitude to all.

Paul H. Ephross

What Happened to Self-Determination?

Saul B. Bernstein

It matters not how strait the gate,
How charged with punishment the scroll,
I am the captain of my fate,
I am the master of my soul.

Charles Ernest Henley

This is a powerful expression of free will and self-determination. "We Shall Overcome" sings confidence in our ability to change individuals, social attitudes and conditions. But literature and songs present many examples to the contrary: Shakespeare's "There is a destiny which shapes our ends, rough hew them as we will," and "Star-crossed Lovers." Folk songs frequently picture people as helpless in the face of forces beyond their control. The lyrics of the song, "Where Have All The Flowers Gone?" with their answer "Blowing In The Wind" suggest an all-powerful destiny.

The determinism free will controversy has been debated for centuries. If all events were predetermined, there would be little point in social work, which is concerned with planned changes in people and in circumstances. We need free will and self-determination, but are they an illusion? Helen Harris Perlman, in a paper entitled "Self-Determination: Reality or Illusion" wrote:

> If I were forced to answer at once the question posed by my title, instead of being given the privilege of meandering toward it, if you demanded of me, "Tell me in ten words or less what your answer is," I would have to say, "I believe self-determination is nine-tenths illusion and one-tenth reality. Therefore I am committed to supporting and enhancing that illusion and also asking the most, the very most, of the exercise of that one-tenth of it that is real, present and possible in our lives." (Perlman, 1967)

Nature and society are replete with illustrations of happenings beyond our control: violent storms, extremes of temperature, wars, droughts, economic depressions and others are "Blowing in the Wind." To say that the predetermined proportion can be reduced to a specific figure such as ninety percent is to be more precise than the facts seem to justify, but certainly events beyond our control loom large and numerous. How we deal with them expresses our self-determination, which applies also to less imposing events.

The question of whether self-determination really exists could be endlessly argued. For me, it makes sense to posit the concept with confidence and to build on it. But just what is it? There are three meanings. It is a fundamental human need. Imagine yourself in a situation, perhaps in prison, in which others decide when you are to get up in the morning, what you are to have for breakfast, the kind of work to do, and on and on, with little or no room for your preferences all through your life. This is a prescription for misery. Valuing of human beings requires rich opportunities for making one's own decisions, whether they are wise or foolish. A society which respects and provides for free decisions, when appropriate, for its citizens is on a high level of desirability and ethics. It is, in fact, a criterion for assessing societies.

A second meaning of self-determination is that it is a value to be honored, providing a philosophic and motivational basis for behavior. As a value, self-determination should guide our thinking and action in our services to people. Various qualifications will be dealt with below.

A third meaning is that it should flow through our methods of working with people. We help clients to make their own decisions, carefully weighing the pros and cons, rather than imposing our ideas on them. Whatever the goals of the service may be, we have learned that it is much more effective and helpful to build on what clients need and want, to take full account of the goals and feelings of our clients, rather than to push hard for what we think is best. It may seem to be feasible to achieve *our* changes, but the result is apt to be conformity rather than internalized change. When the pressure to conform is removed, clients are likely to bounce back to where they were, like a released rubber band. Internalized changes tend to be more abiding.

To examine the complications and qualifications in self-determination, I draw on my article, "Self-Determination: King or Citizen in the Realm of Values" (Bernstein, 1960). I developed the theme in a series of steps:

1. It is the supreme value, to be followed above all others. Social workers would try to satisfy the desires of the group members. This is a simple minded position, which leads to a multitude of difficulties.
2. The wants a person states are often just one side of an ambivalence. Accepting and acting on it as final violates the other side of the ambivalence. Over time, and with the help of the worker and other members, contrary concerns are apt to emerge. All of us have faced decisions laden with pros and cons. An advantage in the group process is for others to express considerations of both sides of the ambivalence. If none of the members do this, the worker can fill the gap.
3. Reality sets limits which are physical, biological, and social. To disregard them is to invite trouble. There is an old maxim about accepting what we cannot change, and making the most of what is flexible.
4. We are each embedded in a complex network of relationships in the group and outside of it. If members yielded entirely to their own impulses, groups could not function. This applies

to all relationships, especially to the more intimate ones, such as the family. Individual drives are strong and need to be modified for the system to flourish. Social hunger is a powerful motivation to join and to be a continuing part of groups. If members insist on their own preferences without regard for those of others, they are likely to lose the opportunities to participate in an enterprise that they need and want. We accept the egocentricity of infants who show no consideration of others. For people older than infants, maturation, perspective on oneself in relation to others, is a long, hard road, but the rewards are great.

5. A more rational and ripened approach which weighs the total situation, including the impact on others, is the goal. A prime purpose of group work is to help members learn how to make intelligent decisions, an ability that will benefit them for the rest of their lives.

Fundamental as self-determination is, it is not the supreme value, the king. Respect for human worth is more important, and when the two are in conflict, the latter should prevail. Fortunately, the two values tend to harmonize, and self-determination is usually an expression of and serves to implement human worth.

Over the years, the great bulk of group work experience has been with people who want to participate in a group. They have had contrary impulses, but the desire to join outweighed the negatives. There have been exceptions, of course. I recall a group in a prison. Various stipulations, such as not being allowed to use sharp tools for arts and crafts, had to be met but the inmates decided whether to join or not and had other choices. In an institution, especially in a prison, where choices are few, the opportunity to make some decisions is sorely needed.

Other examples of limited choices are some groups in psychiatric settings and street work with teenage gangs wherever they congregate. If the gang does not want the worker, they can tell her/him in their own strong street language; more frequently, they just do not appear at the usual place. In the early days of street work, a primary concern was whether the worker could establish a meaningful relationship with the gang. Many experiences have demonstrated success in doing so. A mutually accepted contract, instead of occurring at the very beginning, developed gradually when the members learned through experience that the worker had much to offer them.

In recent years, group work has faced numerous situations in which joining and continuing to attend have been mandated. A judge or someone else in authority ordered participation regardless of the desires of the individuals. The alternative was apt to be going to prison or losing a driver's license. With strong resistance, potential members have joined, regarding this as the lesser of evils.

These conditions have applied especially to alcoholics and other substance abusers. With their long and deep commitment to self-determination, group workers face a difficult choice in such groups. They can refuse to abide by the mandate, but that would cut off the opportunity to be helpful to people who obviously need it. Mostly, they have decided to work within the imposed framework.

This decision carries with it serious problems. Group members are apt to be angry, feeling that a part of their lives is no longer under their own control, and that it is vested in the group and the worker, an enterprise that is undefined for the members at the beginning. Frequent denial of the behavior for which they are being punished adds to the complications. Those who engage in incest are apt to claim that they were merely showing love to the child. Alcoholics may admit to taking a few drinks, but reject being labeled alcoholic. Compounding the problem is the low status of the behavior of which they are accused. A prison chaplain told me that the murderers, robbers and rapists in prison regarded child abusers with horror as the lowest of the low. Alcoholics are not assessed as quite that bad but their status is low. The need for denial is thus reinforced.

Some may find a degree of relief in having an authority make the decision for them, reflecting repressed dissatisfaction with the troubling behavior. They probably have tried to change but failed. Now the choice is forced on them, tying into and supporting whatever feelings they have that want a different kind of life.

Group workers face the complex, lengthy and trying task of helping these individuals move from angry resistance to a stage in which they have come to grips with the destructiveness of their behavior and are enabled to attain control and perspective so that they can diminish or eliminate the impulses leading to it and to face fully the damage they are inflicting on others. The dynamics of this profound change need to be more carefully studied, developing a better understanding for more effective work. Yet, the current state of our knowledge permits and suggests some guidelines. Long experience with a wide variety of groups provides knowledge that at least in part can be applied to mandated groups. The members have needs and characteristics in common with other kinds of people, and much that we have learned is relevant.

Confidentiality should be made part of the contract. Participants should be made aware of the exceptions, such as what the worker is required to report to the court. Anxiety and uncertainty attend the beginnings of practically all groups, and these feelings, including anger, are apt to be more intense in those that are mandated. The worker and the other members are unknowns to each other. Expectations are hazy, with much wondering and concern about how members may be treated.

The worker can offer help to members in the first session by articulating these feelings and showing sympathy with them, not approving the behavior but accepting the person. This could free them to talk about how they feel, an important first step. Moods may be stormy, but the worker should understand that the hostility is directed toward his or her role, not at who the worker really is as a person. Perspective, patience and commitment are required to live through and beyond this turmoil.

Since the members are in the group because of an authoritative decision, they are apt to assume that the worker is part of the corrections system, intent on punishing them. Early in the relationship, the worker should explain that he or she is not working for the corrections department (unless indeed this *is* the case), that the purpose is not to punish but to be helpful to members. There is apt to be skepticism, but with the repetition, time and experience needed to make this position clear, its validity can become convincing.

The fact that members are in effect forced to attend needs to be stated as a reality. But the worker should share with the group that they are free to make the decisions in other areas. Toward the end of the first session, the members might be asked what they would like to discuss at the next meeting. After agreement is reached, specific issues or activities could be suggested for them to think about and do in the interim. There is room for choices by the members in such matters as subjects to be considered, choices about time and place of the meetings. Constant alertness is in order for the worker for issues which can be decided by the members, giving them a basis for feeling that they have some control over what happens in the group, thereby enhancing their self-esteem.

Since the group has been practically forced on the members, their perception of it is apt to be negative and hostile. For constructive change to occur, this feeling must be superseded by one that is friendly, caring, supportive and welcoming to whatever contributions the members are ready to make. When one presents a problem or takes a stand, the worker might ask, "How can we help John with this issue? It seems important to him." As the responses and interactions begin to flow, others may claim the group's attention for what is on their minds. The worker could suggest "These are important too, but let's deal with them after we have discussed John's issue enough to be helpful to him." A danger in group considerations of problems is that of a kind of moving focus, with the result that there is little or no sustained attention to anyone. This could promote both cynicism about the worth of the group and the feeling that no one really cares. Each significant issue should be in focus long enough to reach some type of closure, which could range from a satisfactory resolution, to asking an expert on the subject, to agreement that not enough is known to justify a conclusion. Repeated experiences with hit and run approaches are frustrating. To involve the members in decision making, the worker might ask the one who posed the question and others whether the discussion has gone far enough and whether they are ready for the group to move on.

There could well be "snow-jobbing," saying what the members think the worker wants to hear. If a decision is pending about renewing a driver's license or permission for members to see their children, or anything else important to the members, the temptation to play games is increased. If the worker is required to report to someone in authority about attendance, attitudes and behavior in the group, that fact should be shared with them, emphasizing that the worker understands their feelings, but that he or she is concerned with real change, not with pretty speeches. At times, if a comment is of dubious sincerity, the worker could turn to the others to ask what they think, hoping that one or more of them will be honest. The point is to convey the fact that the worker is not taken in by what is said, without putting down the individual. Humor can help.

Strong defenses create obstacles. But they serve a purpose in the make-up of the personality. Significant change can occur only when defenses are loosened. In a group of alcoholics, a member proclaimed loudly that, although he takes an occasional drink, he is definitely not an alcoholic. Another member, in strong language, pointed out that all of them talked that way, that the previous speaker had better face reality, that he was fooling nobody but himself. Coming from other alcoholics, confrontation is less threatening than if it came from the worker, whose aim is to encourage the group to take responsibility. Recognizing that the self-image of each member is precarious, the worker tries to create a supportive mood so that confrontations are regarded as an expression of caring rather than of attack.

Situations in which members are especially vulnerable to sliding back into the troublesome behavior should be identified and explored. The group can be challenged to think about how such temptations can be handled constructively. Groups often have impressive ideas. Our job is to stimulate them to utilize fully the resources within themselves. Role playing dramatizes the situations, adds a life-like quality to them, providing a good basis for the ensuing discussion.

An objection might be raised to the sympathetic stance in this paper, claiming that those driving under the influence of alcohol and abusers, for example, have hurt people and broken the law. Therefore, they should be punished, going to prison. Certainly, victims, actual or potential, deserve protection against further risks. The alcoholic should not be permitted to drive and the abuser must be separated from his victim. Some should go to prison. But incarceration is expensive, jails are overcrowded, prisoners cannot support their families and fragile egos are further damaged. Such treatment offers little hope for changes in a constructive direction. The aim should rather be to help perpetrators to deal with their unhealthy needs, to build their self-respect, to sensitize them to what they have been doing to others. This approach offers hope.

As with groups generally, a contract is important, indicating the expectations of the worker. Requirements should be clarified. If a court insists on being informed of what goes on in the group, the members should know about it. (The worker should argue against this stipulation with the referring court, trying to keep the demands to a minimum.) Other expectations of the members need to be made clear.

The members are apt to find it difficult at the beginning to formulate their part of the contract, but as the group develops, they should be encouraged to express their goals. They have a heavy investment in the enterprise and deserve an opportunity to build in their preferences. They should also know the areas in which they are free to make decisions.

The treatment of sex abuse provides illustrations of many of these points. Henry Giaretto of San Jose, California, has developed a comprehensive program for serving sex abusers, their victims, their families and others. The over-all title of the program is Parents United. A sponsor from the agency meets each new person and invites her/him to a Pre-orientation Group, where the welcome is warm and supportive. There are then Parenting Groups, one for Daughters and Sons, one for Family Reconstruction Strategy, for Alcoholics, a group for those speaking only Spanish, a group for Adults Molested as Children, a sexuality class at a nearby university; Making Life Happen Your Way for ages 18 to 25, and individual counseling are both offered. People who have lived through and profited from the above serve as volunteer group leaders and counselors. The emphasis is on trying to keep families together and on providing support and hope.

This program seems to show good results, and Parents United has spread to a large number of places. Printed material and training are available at their headquarters. Unfortunately the group process and methods are not fully described or analyzed, but there is much to be learned from Parents United.

Mothers in families in which their husbands are involved with their daughters are in a traumatic and puzzling situation. The wife is fearful about destroying the family and threatening their income if her husband is reported to the police and possibly sent to prison. In one group, a statement was made that the mothers always know about the incest. One woman protested hotly that it went on in her family a long time before she found out about it. Living with this welter of complications, mothers need help, and a group is a good means for providing it.

The daughters are also in a difficult position, when they realize that sexual activity with their fathers or other adult males is not normal or socially healthy. She faces the warnings the abuser gave her if she tells anyone, it will endanger the family, he may go to jail, and he will not be able to continue to support the family. He may also threaten violence. All of this is a heavy load and the youngster may postpone telling anyone about it for a long time. If she informs her mother, she could be accused of lying or of encouraging her father sexually. Groups for these girls are very much in order.

Former victims of incest, even if it occurred long ago, need help. In a first session of a group with this background, the worker said that all of them had been victims, and she hoped that they would gain a great deal from each other. An audible sigh went through the room. Each was no longer alone in her misery, feeling that she was practically the only one carrying this burden of a painful memory. As they talked, it became clear that they thought of themselves as soiled, as pariahs, as somewhat responsible for the incest. The group helped them realize that they were not responsible for the incest, that they need no longer carry the burden of guilt, and that they were entitled to a much improved image of themselves.

An important goal with former victims and others is a balanced view of males. This is especially urgent with battered women. If the agency is aggressively anti-male, the clients are apt to develop a stereotype of men, that they are all like the batterer. Whatever may be the future course of the lives of these women, males are certain to figure in them. Allowing a generous amount of time in groups for the women to express their feelings about the men who exploited and abused them, attention might then be turned toward other points of view. Not all men are like the ones who made them suffer, nor are they all alike. The group can help in thinking about relationships with the other sex that are mutually respecting. Ways of finding out whether a man really cares for one should be explored, as well as the qualities of genuinely reciprocal relationships with males.

To stimulate and support this approach, the agency needs to have a balanced point of view. As is true of other minorities, who have been victimized, overreaction is understandable. This has happened with Jews, blacks and others. In the long run, a more rational stance is needed to enable the victims to achieve satisfying relationships.

In working with the men, the wives, and the children, it is desirable to form groups for each category separately. Feelings are apt to be strong and confrontations at the beginning between perpetrators and victims and wives could easily go out of control. After they have attained some perspective in their separate groups, mixing members is apt to be more productive. At the early stages, they need the support and insights of others like themselves so they will feel free to give full expression to the turmoil within. Later, they are in a better position to deal with the other categories. That the abusers and their families know that all of them are in groups, should be reassuring to each.

For example, Parents United brings daughters into groups of male perpetrators not including their own fathers. The girls make clear to the men what incest did to them. (For the sake of simplicity in presentation, I have not referred to male boyfriends of mothers, uncles, grandfathers and male victims. Points made above might have to be adjusted to fit each of these categories.)

Alcoholics have Alcoholics Anonymous and their families are served by Al-Anon. Both are widely available. There are numerous other organizations that work with alcoholics. Those referred by courts provide opportunities for group workers to give service. For those considering moving in this direction, it is essential to have a clear understanding with the courts about the expectations on both sides. A key issue is whether it is expected to share with the court personnel what is said in meetings with clients. It would be much better to be able to maintain confidentiality. If group workers are considering other kinds of work with alcoholics, a careful review of those available is in order.

Moving into service to abusers and alcoholics by group work faces the stubborn obstacles of limited budgets and staff. The use of carefully selected and trained volunteers, part-time workers and paraprofessionals would increase our resources and it has been done extensively in the past. Co-leaders have worked with trained workers, providing an opportunity for effective supervision, preparing supervisees for more independent practice in the future. Parents United uses former members of abuser groups as co-leaders in new groups. A thoughtful assessment of the qualifications and readiness of the individual is essential. This could be a good resource for staff.

Over the years of group work's history, group workers have been responsive to human needs as illustrated by expanded practice in psychiatric settings, homes for unmarried mothers, teenage gangs, parents of victims of homicide, and many, many others. Child abuse and alcoholism create intense misery and challenge us to provide groups for helping. Our knowledge and skill can offer hope, especially in the way we free and stimulate members to help each other. The mandated aspect complicates the situation, but it does provide a potential point of contact. Experience shows that many people in the serious predicament of abuse and alcoholism can be reached and helped. Despite the loss of self-determination at the beginning, we can still call upon this concept in the course of the development of the group. Moving towards self-determination has the inestimable advantage of building on the strengths of the members, their healthy and self-respecting impulses, and this is a major step on the road to maturity in human relations.

REFERENCES

Bernstein, S. 1960. "Self-Determination: King or Citizen in the Realm of Values," *Social Work*, (January).

Giaretto, H. 1982. *Integrated Treatment of Child Sexual Abuse: A Treatment and Training Manual*, Science and Behavior Books, Palo Alto, California.

Perlman, H. 1967. "Self-Determination: Reality or Illusion," in *Values in Social Work: A Re-examination*, Monograph IX, National Association of Social Workers.

The Rediscovery of Real-World Groups

Paul H. Ephross
Thomas V. Vassil

INTRODUCTION

This discussion deals with the sociology of group work knowledge by examining what the intellectual tradition of group work has to say about groups composed of citizens, professionals, legislators and administrators: "real-world" groups. Such groups are formed in order to produce a product other than simply changes in their members. Others have referred to these as "taskgroups," "administrative groups," "working groups," or "groups that work" (Ephross and Vassil, 1988). Mills (1984) has referred to their purposes as "the pursuit of a collective goal." Many such groups, boards and commissions and their sub-units, for example, have fiduciary or statutory responsibility for the governance of agencies and organizations. Other real-world groups express the desires of their members for social and/or political change and accomplishment. Still others express the agendas of memberships defined by their ethnic or racial identities, their geographical origins or locations, or their age-groups or work affiliations. Staff groups certainly fall within our purview here.

Focusing on such groups does not in any way seek to disparage the meaning and value of groups formed for other purposes. Both groups formed for clinical treatment and those formed for the education and socialization of their members deserve the attention they have received and should continue to receive. Skill in working with them and the empirical knowledge on which such skill should increasingly be based are important topics for group workers' attention. This discussion restricts itself to real-world groups because they have not received the attention they deserve in recent decades (Ephross, 1986).

The reasons for this comparative neglect are both apparent and elusive at the same time. Working groups are important in their members' lives. Within social work, for example, as we have pointed out elsewhere,

> . . . some of the events that are most important . . . take place within working groups. Points of view are accepted or rejected. Decisions are reached which either enable and support, or frustrate and disparage the deepest purposes of professions, organizations, and individuals. Organizations, services, agencies and projects are funded or ended as a result of decisions reached in groups. Particular targets of services are selected. Criteria for future decisions are developed . . . Judgements are made, hirings and firings planned and confirmed, influence strategies adopted, and rewards and sanctions distributed, all within the context of working groups in which professionals serve as members, chairs, staff, or sometimes all three. (Ephross and Vassil, 1988, p. 2)

So it is all the more puzzling that group work has gone through a period of neglect of such groups. It is important to understand some of the reasons why group workers–some, certainly not all–colluded to neglect an important aspect of their own history and intellectual tradition. This is our first task. Second, we shall look at a central dialectical tension in real-world groups which we think is vital for understanding, working in, and learning more about such groups. Finally, we shall suggest an avenue for returning working groups to the forefront of attention, not only for group workers, (where they would only be returning to their original place of importance) but also for the entire social work profession and, indeed, for a broader audience as well.

It is tempting, especially under the auspices of an organization which owes its origin to a commemoration of the genius of Grace Coyle, to point out that she knew and wrote sixty years ago some of what we are going to say (Coyle, 1930). There is a great deal of truth to such an observation. She did, and so did others of our intellectual forebears and teachers, such as William Schwartz (1976), Alan Klein (1953), Gertrude Wilson and Gladys Ryland (1949). Group work should celebrate its origins, to be sure, but also needs to move on and continue to regain its place at the leading edge of the rapidly evolving social work profession in a period of accelerating social change.

THE DEMOCRATIC MICROCOSM
AND THE BUREAUCRATIZED SOCIETY

One of the central questions for what is left of the twentieth century is how to get any large service-delivery system to work right. This is a problem for all large systems in all fields of human endeavor, nowhere more so than in the management of social services. There is an enormous proliferation of books which essentially and unanimously critique existing models of management. Whether they recommend management by walking around, by targeting minutes, by establishing quality circles, or by installing changed organizational cultures, virtually all critics attack the results of locking people into rigid, bureaucratically ordered structures. Within such structures higher and higher levels of work–some of it in the range of what has been considered professional work–is commoditized, mechanized, its outputs weighed and counted, its technologies routinized, its qualities judged by statistical tests whose assumptions are not fulfilled by the situations in which they are used.

Strangely enough, in social work such distortions have increased as social work has become steadily more important to the broader society. As we have moved further and further out of our former obscurity and into the mainstream of public concern, the same distortions which originated in industry and government have been applied to social work. The trouble is that such approaches to getting organizations to work well didn't work elsewhere, and certainly don't work in social agencies and other service delivery organizations. In her brilliant book, Systems Concepts and Public Policy, Ida Hoos has suggested that the philosophical and intellectual constructs on which management-by-systems-concepts are based are just incompatible with both the goals and the processes of public policy-based service delivery. Hoos paints on a broad canvas, but her observations are important for social work as well. Systems-based approaches, themselves originally intended as an antidote to the failures of heavy-handed formal bureaucracies to stay in touch with their external and internal environments, tend to succumb to the same fatal flaws they were intended to remedy, she argues.

A competing view of organizational structure–one deeply rooted in group work's past–is that of a democratic microcosm. Each of these two words deserves close attention. By "democratic" we mean a group which has progressed far enough through the processes of group formation that it is real and salient as a symbolic entity in the lives of its members. In a democratic group, the rules of civility, commitment and equanimity have been brought into being through the shared experiences and developed commitments of its members. In such a group, the tension between cohesion and conflict which will be discussed below provides a motive which leads to task accomplishment and group growth rather than fear, distrust, and danger. A democratic group is a place of both safety and challenge for its members.

The term "microcosm," literally means small world. This view of a group was the vision that informed much of group work history. It was derived from the insights of Dewey (1939) and Follett (1930), Lindeman (1924) and Lewin (1951). The idea of a democratic microcosm implies that the larger society is built of smaller sub-units. It connotes the need for human beings to learn democracy, a respect for differences, commitment, civility, how to deal with conflict, and the dynamics of task accomplishments in small settings so that they can be applied in larger organizations and in communities. The concept does not deny the differences between the small and the informal, on the one hand, and the large, formal organization on the other, but it traces a continuity between the two. In short, the concept of democratic microcosms in group updates, focuses, and applies to real-world groups what was once referred to as a "social goals" view of the purposes of group work (Klein, 1972).

What, one may ask, is so wonderful about a group, specifically a working group, which is a democratic microcosm? It has three characteristics which make it invaluable, because such a group may be viewed as a complete, though always imperfect system. First, it has gyroscopic abilities in relation to its external environment. Its internal climate of democracy and valued participation operate to prevent the group from going too far out of equilibrium with its external environment, and its admission of deviant points of view exerts a similar influence inside the group. Second, because a democratic microcosm attracts the commitment of its members, it can manufacture from within its membership the roles which it needs in order to accomplish its tasks. Third, it provides an ongoing learning laboratory for its members, and thus accomplishes an educational function for the society which other social institutions either neglect or take for granted. A person whose education has not included learning within the framework of democratic microcosms will be all too ready to accept stultifying bureaucracy as the natural order of mass communications and mindless conformity as the natural order of the social contract. On the other hand, democratic microcosms can be viewed as extremely threatening by bureaucratic organizations. This sense of threat is often manifested by artificially dividing group tasks dichotomously into task and process, external and internal, public and private, or even into a barely disguised dualism of masculine and feminine. Group workers have long known that effective work in groups requires both a warm heart and a cool head, simultaneously, and that dichotomous formulations do not reflect the ways tasks are accomplished in real-world groups.

We much prefer the monistic view of the relationship between task accomplishment and socio-emotional processes argued by Bales (1970), Schwartz (1976), Thelen (1981), and by Schon in his reflections on how professionals relate to interpersonal processes (1983). Such a view also fits the experiences of generations of practitioners in groups because of the social values which are immanent in it. In order for groups to accomplish tasks they, as well as the professionals who staff them, need to deal simultaneously with process and product, task system and socio-emotional system, order and disorder. To try to separate these elements is to deny the essence of what happens in groups.

THE DIALECTICAL RELATIONSHIP BETWEEN COHESION AND CONFLICT

What, then, do we know about working groups? We know two salient aspects which need to guide our practice with such groups.

These are the principles of civility and commitment to the group itself, and the positive values for group development of the tension between cohesion and conflict in groups. Each has major implications both for practice in real-world groups and teaching others skills in this practice.

Much of what passes for professional leadership in working groups–whether from the status of staff ("worker") or from the status of chair–can be viewed as more negative than positive in its effects on group development and group growth. We base this observation not only on our own experience but on many years of working with students and staffs in the roles of teachers and consultants. Working groups can be prevented from completing the processes of group formation and their processes subverted by a variety of behaviors. Often these are consciously motivated, to be sure, on the part of the group's leadership lest groups, once formed, become forces for change within their larger organizations. Sometimes these behaviors are unwitting. Staffs provide the most glaring examples, but there is no lack of other examples to be gleaned from a review of meetings of boards, commissions, committees, inter-agency task forces and many other kinds of groups. Using meeting times to communicate material which can better be processed in written form, subversion of decision-making processes, spending time in allocating faults rather than in engaging in problem-solving processes constitute only a partial list of behaviors which prevent group formation and group productivity. To enjoy the benefits of group processes and group decision-making, the development of a group needs to be fostered rather than prevented.

A productive group is characterized, in our view, by an ongoing dynamic and productive tension between cohesion and conflict. For learning to take place in a group, the members need an atmosphere of civility and safety. Such an atmosphere can arise only within a framework of unconditional regard for the integrity of the group. Unconditional regard does not imply false agreement, nor does it by any means imply a reluctance to engage in conflict and processes of dealing with this conflict. In fact, the very gyroscopic forces which were referred to above require a conscious willingness to allow, indeed at times to encourage, the expression of minority opinions, thus surfacing rather inhibiting conflict.

Both cycles, those of cohesion and conflict, are important in the development of the group. Cohesion fosters psychological safety, dependability and foresight. It provides a basis for self-esteem. Closeness also generates conflict because the safer people feel, the freer they are to raise annoying issues. And these produce disconfirmations, which mean trouble.

Conflict produces unpredictability, uncertainty, and anxiety. At the same time it can produce more scouting behavior by the group, expand the search for alternatives, and sharpen the focus on issues. Bonds of closeness can contain the extent of the conflict even while generating it. Both cycles, in our point of view, are necessary. The trick is to develop in the group the ability to work under stress. Work means the more interpersonal exchange of ideas, feelings, skills, and motivations.

In our view, these demands call for a practitioner who has a broad range of knowledge of skills that includes the abilities to recognize problems and determine issues, seek pertinent data, set forth courses of action, work with people, reach reasonable decisions under pressure of time and control and evaluate performance. Worker qualities such as perseverance, imagination, courage, and flexibility are also needed. Professionals who staff working groups need to be tough minded problem solvers who, in their work, do not seek a fixed reality but rather approach tasks in the context of the discipline and art of practice. They have to be people who can deal with the tensions between what they know and don't know in a time-oriented, task-specific framework. In more abstract terms the professional function in groups places social work practitioners squarely in the context of the pushes and pulls between order and disorder which resonate in a continuous and uneasy balance. The concept of equanimity captures the ability of the professional to keep the good and the bad in reasonable balance.

Safety for group members depends on unconditional regard for the group taking first place over the momentary tensions and anger which can accompany conflict. Group members' anxieties are held in check by this unconditional regard, so that the commitment to the group, which arises from cohesion, can allow group members to be comfortable with conflict. The book needs to be given more importance than the candle, as it were; the development of a mature group needs to be given more importance than specific decisions by the group or positions taken by individual members. Membership in a real-world group includes two commitments: to engage in conflict and decision-making, and to do so within an overall framework of civility. Lacking either of these commitments, or given a climate which makes either impossible, what results is a non-group, or what can be called a "groupoid." It looks like a group, at least at times, and it may even sound like a group, but it doesn't produce the benefits of a group, and in the long run its members lack commitment to it.

Does this abstract discussion sound impractical? Quite to the contrary, it is only when careful attention has been paid to these variables that groups can truly achieve the practical purposes for which they are intended. Paralleling Lewin's oft-quoted aphorism that nothing is as practical as a good theory, nothing is as valuable to an organization as a staff, a board, or a committee or commission which has developed into a fully-formed group. Attention and patience devoted to the processes of group formation can pay direct and measurable dividends for an organization both in the commitment of the members to the purposes of the group and the development of a constituency of friends and supporters of the organization. It is precisely because the organizational environment sometimes feels like "a jungle out there" that attention needs to be paid to group development "in here": that is, within the structure of the organization. Phrased in familiar group work terms, it is exactly when the product is important that the most attention needs to be paid to the processes.

One may object to this point of view. Our society has come to accept a sort of corporate model of leadership, one in which policy-making boards are sometimes listed on letterheads but really are viewed as willing to engage in some of the demanding processes sketched above. Both industry and government have often ignored the requirements for group development in the course of the pressures of day-to-day organizational survival and operation. This observation explains some of the problems which have beset both. The fascination with other nations' management systems, clouded and confused though it often is with a variety of political and ideological baggage, contains an awareness that somehow they seem to have achieved better production by paying more attention to working group processes.

Is there anything new in focusing on the reciprocal relationship between cohesion in groups and their development of a capacity to deal with conflict? Here again we need to return to the roots of our group work learnings. Our observations are very much in the spirit of Lewin's "unfreezing-learning-refreezing" paradigm (1951) and Glidewell's scheme of the process of change and growth (1975). Additional conceptual points of view in this discussion are related to Benne's observation that group members need help in avoiding polarities so that they can devote energy to reconciling paradoxes in the course of group life.

LEARNING AND TEACHING ABOUT REAL-WORLD GROUPS

In the course of advanced education in social work–with a concentration in social group work, let it be noted–one of us once had occasion to consult the card catalogue of the great Boston Public Library. On a whim, he looked in the catalogue for "Social Group Work." There was no such card. For a moment, a feeling of doubt crept over him. What did it mean to be enrolled in a graduate degree program in the field so obscure that it was not even known to one of the world's great storehouses of knowledge? Perhaps the thing to do was to transfer to casework? A helpful librarian solved the problem. The heading under which to look was entitled, "Group Work, Educational and Social." With a sigh of relief, he was able to find the object of his search, and begin a process of study which still engages him today.

The point of this reminiscence is that different generations and different societies package knowledge under different labels. In our age of computerized data bases, it may be more timely to refer to this phenomenon in contemporary terms: various data bases bound and arrange their sub-sets differently. Suppose that much of the content of this discussion up to this point is today considered part of management rather than group work. Does this distinction make a difference? Should one be concerned about the labels if the bottle's contents are the same? Some would argue that one should not, that an attachment to traditional terms such as group work cloud the issue, and prevent the broader fields of social work and the cognate human service professions from being able to learn and utilize knowledge about work in and with groups.

This is a defensible position. But after years of trying to integrate content such as that presented in this discussion with other methods and processes, it is the conclusion of the writers that group work, particularly group work with real-world groups, deserves and requires both emphasis and a degree of separateness in order to be learned and taught effectively. Its origins are unique. It's conceptual base is in the sociology and social psychology of small groups, as well as in the practice wisdom of early group work pioneers. Its research needs at this point in its history are particular and marked (Ephross & Vassil, Ch. 12). Its applicability and value, for social workers and many others, remains broad and deep.

For both students and practitioners, the rediscovery of real-world groups can have particular importance. Reaffirming the validity of work in groups, participation, investment of self and commitment to building effective group structures can provide social workers with tools of affirmation and with tools of effectiveness. It can also help to build organizations that work, and to provide organizational atmospheres which prevent the practice of social work from becoming dehumanized.

REFERENCES

Bales, R.F. 1970. *Personality and Interpersonal Behavior.* New York: Holt, Rinehard, and Winston.

Benne, K.D. 1964. From polarization to Paradox. In L.P. Bradford, J.R. Gibb, and K.D. Benne, eds. *T. Group Theory and Laboratory Method.* New York: John Wiley.

Coyle, G.L. 1930. *Social Process in Organized Groups.* New York: Richard R. Smith.

Dewey, J. 1939. *Experience and Education.* New York: Macmillan.

Ephross, P.H. 1986. Group work with work groups: a case of arrested development. In P.H. Glasser and N.S. Mayadas, eds. *Group Workers at Work: Theory and Practice for the '80s.* Totowa, NJ: Rowman and Littlefield.

Ephrass, P.H. and T.V. Vassil. *Groups That Work.* NY Columbia University Press, 1988.

Follett, M.P. 1930. A social psychology of laboratory training. In K.D. Benne et al., *The Laboratory Method of Changing and Learning*. Palo Alto, CA: Science and Behavior Books.

Glidewell, J. 1975. A Social Psychology of Laboratory Training. In K.D. Benne et al., eds. *The Laboratory Method of Changing and Learning*. Palo Alto, CA: Science and Behavior Books.

Hoos, I.R. 1983. *Systems Analysis in Public Policy: A Critique*, Revised ed., Berkeley: University of California Press.

Klein, A.F. 1953. Society–Democracy–and the Group. New York: Whiteside, Morrow.

Klein, A.F. 1972. *Effective Groupwork: An Introduction to Principle and Method.* New York: Association Press.

Lewin, K. 1951. *Field Theory in Social Science*. New York: Harper & Row.

Lindeman, E. 1924. *Social Discovery*. New York: Republic Books.

Mills, T.M. 1984. *The Sociology of Small Groups*, 2nd ed. Englewood Cliffs, NJ: Prentice-Hall.

Oichi, W.G. 1984. *Theory Z*. Reading, MA: Addison-Wesley.

Peters, T.J. and R.H. Waterman. 1982. *In Search of Excellence: Lessons from America's Best-Run companies*. New York: Harper & Row.

Schon, D. 1983. *The Reflective Practitioner*. New York: Basic Books.

Schwartz, W. 1976. Between client and system: the mediating function. In R. Roberts and H. Northen, eds. *Theories of Social Work with Groups*. New York: Columbia University Press.

Thelen, H.A. 1981. *The Classroom Society*. New York: Halsted Press.

Wilson, G. and G. Ryland. 1949. *Social Group Work Practice*. Cambridge, MA: Houghton Mifflin.

Confronting Human Finitude:
Group Work with People with AIDS

George S. Getzel
Kevin F. Mahony

This paper represents the cumulative experience of a support group for gay men with AIDS which began in May, 1986 and which continues to meet every Monday from 6:00 to 7:30 p.m. at Gay Men's Health Crisis in New York City. Three group leaders and 27 members have contributed their time and their energies through fair weather and in the bitterest winter. Of the 27 men who have at one time or another been members of the group, the oldest is 63 years old, and the youngest (who died last January) was 25. Eight men in varying degrees of health currently remain in the group. Over the course of the last 2 1/2 years, 11 have died and 2 have gone home to their families during the final stages of their illness. Two men remained in the group for less than 2 months, and 4 dropped out after approximately six months for a variety of reasons which they were encouraged to share with the group. The leadership of the group has also changed somewhat over the past 2 1/2 years. One of the original co-leaders (Richard Gambe), who had already been diagnosed with AIDS when the group began, decided it was time for him to leave in November of 1987. His replacement (Kevin Mahony), who began with this group in December of 1987, was himself diagnosed with AIDS in January of 1988, and continues as co-leader.

The significance and power of the group for all of its members at the time of their participation, however brief or extended that time might be, cannot be overemphasized. Even when they could not attend because of severe illness or hospitalization, members told us that they would recall the time and place of the meeting, in an effort to reach the turbulent, life-giving atmosphere of the group. Some men who have dropped out still maintain contact with the workers and ask about other members of the group. Members of the group visit one another in the hospital, have dinner or go out for drinks and an evening at the opera together, and attend a relentless series of funerals and memorial services–the tribal rituals of life in the time of AIDS.

We dedicate this paper to those 27 men who have affected our own lives immeasurably, and whose lives we hope we have enriched through our efforts. Although we have shared some painful moments, the paradox of this work is that this group has given us a heightened sense of the preciousness of life and the need, as Martin Buber says, of "an I for a thou." We are committed to helping the group maintain lives of quality and meaning, in whatever terms each person defines it, and much of our philosophy of group work with Persons with AIDS (PWAs) can be epitomized in this quote from the playwright William Saroyan: "In the time of your life, live–so that in that wondrous time you shall not add to the misery and sorrow of the world, but shall smile at the infinite delight and mystery of it."

From the beginning of the AIDS epidemic, group work has been seen as a valuable modality to help PWAs overcome social isolation and gain some measure of control over their destinies; throughout the country, hundreds of such groups meet weekly. Their continuing existence attests to participants' strong needs to universalize sometimes overwhelming emotional responses to the stresses of this devastating disease, to problem-solve around strategies for coping with its effects, and to exchange resources which can enhance the quality of an uncertain and abbreviated life.

In an earlier paper, Gambe and Getzel (1988) suggested guidelines for group composition, co-leadership and interventive strategies for PWA groups during different phases of group development. This group work model proposed the following objectives expressed in the actions of the workers and, most important, in the mutual aid process of the membership. The universality of experience which has been identified by Yalom (1985) a therapeutic factor in groups helps to accomplish these objectives: (1) identifying ways for members to reach out to families, friends and lovers for instrumental assistance and emotional support; (2) expressing otherwise unacceptable feelings of rage, sadness, guilt, fear and shame occasioned by different biopsychosocial crises; (3) focusing on the present, and exploring options which may enhance the daily quality of life, both physical and psychological; (4) finding ways to demonstrate care for peers, family and friends who may themselves have become estranged or overwhelmed due to their own fears and anxieties; (5) exploring quality of life issues (how people want to live and, ultimately, to die) as they grow more dependent on others or more disabled; (6) providing positive reinforcement for each member's unique experience as a gay man and a person with AIDS in a society which increasingly exhibits intense homophobia and AIDS-phobia.

These objectives focus on problem-solving of shared concerns through group discussion. Group members can gain a more positive sense of themselves as proactive and empowered, rather than helpless, stigmatized victims of an uncontrollable disease and societal bigotry. Although the problem-solving approach is crucial to giving members a sense of control, another significant facet of the group experience needs to be emphasized: interventions must strategically address the existential questions of the meaning of the disease, suffering and death of PWAs. The multi-level significance of the themes of separation, loss and transcendence is a pervasive subtext of the content and interaction of groups of people with AIDS.

Separation and loss have long been recognized as difficult issues for professionals when they arise within social work practice with individuals, families and groups. Group workers serving PWAs typically share these overwhelming burdens, as they too witness the mounting toll of illness, disability and death among the membership and outside the group. In the short run, group workers' psychological survival and ability to serve this population may be greatly dependent on their capacity for denial of some of the more terrifying aspects of AIDS, and mitigation of the unbearable stresses experienced by the group collectively and individually. However, PWAs may not be fully served as a consequence of this attitude, and ultimately workers may pay a heavy price in cumulative stress, depression and ultimate emotional burnout if they themselves become immersed in this denial (Lopez and Getzel, 1987).

We strongly believe that the skills of the group workers and the group experience can provide significant resources to assist people with AIDS develop their own unique approaches to these powerful questions of personal mortality. Although this is difficult and demanding on the workers as well as the group, the benefits achieved may be extraordinarily meaningful, and filled with hope. As medical technology begins to make advances in the treatment of clinical issues associated with HIV infection, so these groups are helping people to live fuller and richer lives despite the presence of a life-threatening disease, and to find help through a concerned community's support.

In this paper, we will look at the psychosocial responses of people with AIDS to the multiple stressors associated with the disease, and relate them to group development theory. Through practice examples, group work interventions that assist PWAs to cope with these concerns will be identified, and the implications of these practice approaches will be analyzed.

PSYCHOSOCIAL RESPONSES TO AIDS

As Gillian Walker (1987) discusses in writing on AIDS and Family Therapy, it is crucial that workers understand as fully as possible the wide spectrum of human situations which face individuals diagnosed with AIDS, and the severe social and psychological crises which may threaten to overwhelm them as well as their significant others. Needless to say, every individual responds differently to the stresses of living with HIV and AIDS, yet while the diverse populations currently coping with these issues may be vastly different in experience, education level and life-style, some overriding experiences and responses may be common to all.

A sense of helplessness may precede the development of any symptom of opportunistic infections among people who are vulnerable or at risk of an AIDS diagnosis. Respiratory infections, skin rashes, sleeplessness and transitory fevers are a few of the physical symptoms which may be accompanied by psychosomatic symptoms and obsessive thinking (Lopez and Getzel, 1984; 1987; Getzel, 1987). Panicky reactions build if a person has night sweats, swollen glands, weight loss and other symptoms frequently related to HIV infection. Paradoxically, some of this panic may subside once a person develops an opportunistic infection and is given a diagnosis of full-blown AIDS; some people have expressed a sense of emotional relief upon finally "being told what's wrong with me," and for some, the certainty may be easier to manage than the ever-present question: "When is the axe going to fall?" Needless to say, this relief is only temporary as further biological and psychosocial stressors accompany further progression of the disease. The axe, it seems, is always there.

Preoccupation with illness may result in separation from significant persons in a PWA's life, and increasing social isolation although many find renewed or expanded sources of support as their families of origin or their lovers and friends (what we like to think of as their families of choice) rally around the PWA. People with AIDS may come to see themselves as toxic, stigmatized outcasts. Families and friends, who withdraw out of inappropriate fear of infection or moralistic judgments that are frequently attached to a sexually transmitted disease, can exacerbate this sense of stigmatization, and may contribute to the PWA becoming more emotionally withdrawn, depressed, and overwhelmed with feelings of hopelessness and guilt. Health and social service providers, who unfortunately may be equally or even more judgmental, also may act aversive and incite depressive feelings and loss of esteem. Alan related to the group his experience with a nurse whose hostile and insensitive attitude toward him almost led to his stopping the monthly transfusions which he desperately needed. "I always get the feeling she'd rather see me dead," he told the group.

PWAs may experience shame at being exposed as gay or drug users, or sexually linked to these populations. Self-blame is not uncommon as PWAs may bargain to go "straight" or deny their identity as gay men in search of a magical "cure." "If only I hadn't spent so much time having sex, I might not be in this situation today," is the kind of statement that exemplifies this guilt-ridden self-recrimination. In addition, PWAs may feel guilty about the burdens they are placing on others for their care.

Sadness and depression reflect, in part, grief over actual bodily and functional losses. The prospect of dying from AIDS at an age when most people are just beginning to live may open up memories of past losses, such as the death of friends and kin–it is not uncommon for men in these groups to have suffered the loss of a lover and numerous other friends. As Bart once remarked, "Everyone around me is dead and dying–why should I go on living?" Because of the progressive nature of the disease, the seeming irreversibility of the condition, and the often painful and disfiguring deterioration that may occur, some people may contemplate suicide.

In the face of these ultimate questions of living and dying in what is rightly perceived as an increasingly hostile environment, PWAs still have remarkable capacities for hope and optimism, sentiments which are often voiced in the group. Hope is supported when PWAs are enabled to see that life can still have quality and value, and goals (even if short-term ones) can still be attained. In the course of this group, members have started advanced degree programs, taken on new and challenging jobs, moved to new apartments, and found new friends and lovers. Somehow the life force continues to thrive in the death-laden atmosphere of AIDS.

The potency of the group as an antidote to the negative stresses of AIDS increases as the group becomes a safe environment to discuss issues of separation and loss, while serving as a partial substitute for lost or nonexistent social supports. Shared experience is a focus for discussing issues of human finitude in a secure and, in the best of times, nonjudgmental atmosphere. The skills of the group workers and the special power and scope of the phases of group development encourage this process. "Sometimes this feels like the only family we have," Bart once remarked. The group and the workers nodded in agreement.

RELEVANT THEORY

Group development theory affords a useful structure to understand some of the many issues which arise in groups of people with AIDS. Heap (1977) notes that social work groups confront the practitioner with the reality of rapid and dramatic changes requiring an understanding of the cumulative sequence of events, in order to respond to emerging needs and demands in the group. Sequential patterns emerge in the group related to "dependency, identification, relationship, values and goals. As with the individual, these maturational tasks generate internal tension, conflict and defense; the resolution of these is decisive for the group's harmony and efficiency–perhaps for its survival."

When a group such as this anticipates or actually experiences the loss of one or more members due to illness, geographic dislocation or death, the very existence of the group may be threatened and the remaining members' sense of well-being severely tested. Northen (1988) writes that as a group faces termination "the socioemotional issues become separation and coming to terms with the meaning that the group experience has had for the members. The members exhibit anxiety about separation and ambivalence about the loss of relationships with the social worker and other members."

Garland, Jones and Kolodny's model (1965) for stages of group development is rich in the description of the ending or separation phase. It notes that the separation stage has such interactional characteristics as denial, simple regression, regressive, fugue, recapitulation, evaluation, nihilistic flight and positive flight. An understanding of these dynamics may cue the workers as to what is occurring in the group and what are effective strategies for intervention. A separation stage in PWA groups is evoked when there are a significant number of absences or the death of a member. Also the changing of seasons, holidays, such as Christmas and Easter, anniversaries of the deaths of loved ones or the anniversary of one's AIDS diagnosis become highly evocative of separation stage patterns of content and interaction in the group. For example, two men somewhat ruefully recalled that their AIDS diagnoses coincided with the date the Challenger exploded.

Every skill the worker can muster may be called into play as members in the separation phase deal simultaneously with issues of historical and current losses, and concerns about their own potential mortality. It is poignant to note group members grappling with these existential questions with considerable feeling and depth of response while striving to live as fully and normally as possible. Perhaps one is somehow less afraid to die if one is not afraid to live.

Group Illustrations

The following practice excerpts illustrate the separation stage of PWA groups. The dynamic patterns described are not lock-step, but oscillate over a particular session or several sessions. The coworkers systematically engage members at each sub-stage of separation by recognizing the dynamic characteristics occurring in the group.

Denial

Members exhibit simple denial when absences, departures, hospitalizations and even deaths are seemingly forgotten or disregarded. Members may cluster together with a renewed sense of closeness, unconsciously attempting to fill a void in the group with remaining members, or they may further isolate themselves and simply refuse to participate in the discussion.

The workers told the group of unexpectedly receiving a phone call from Ben's mother to say that he had died a week after returning home to Ohio. Alan, a member who had visited Ben almost daily during his last hospitalization in New York said, with muted anger, that he was not surprised Ben had died because he did not take care of himself and was resigned to dying. Alan, a 43-year old gay man who is estranged from his wife and 15-year old daughter, angrily spoke of Ben's family as "too possessive and ignorant about AIDS treatments." Alan's bristling tone was paradoxically accompanied by his telling the group that Ben's parents had thanked him for his assistance.

Not surprisingly, much of the information shared involves discussions of medical treatments, since many group members frequently have a greater amount of medical sophistication than some of their health care providers. While this sharing of information is a valuable and positive function of the group, some members may overemphasize discussions of medical tests and procedures as a way of avoiding disturbing emotional issues. Following Alan's heated response detailed above, the group (led by one member who almost obsessively focuses on highly technical medical information) took off on a discussion of various treatments, rather than helping Alan deal with his anger at Ben's parents, and perhaps at Ben. During a moment of silence in the group, one worker noted that members had grieved the deaths of so many friends and loved ones, and that it is hard for the group when a member dies. The strained silence deepened. The worker mentioned that Ben's family wanted to hold a memorial service in New York at a later date. At this point, Warren asked the group if he could talk about his efforts to get a part-time job, which the group again seized upon eagerly. Two weeks later, Greg (who had been largely silent during the discussion of Ben's death) organized some of the group members (including Alan) to make a panel in Ben's honor for the Names Project Quilt.

Regression

Mounting tensions in a PWA group may be expressed in powerful schismatic exchanges between members who are immersed in their own personal grief. Group conflict is a useful method in displacing anger while masking pervasive depression and sadness. The group may become frozen in conflict as members exhibit hysterical fugue-like behaviors while they unconsciously and symbolically act-out past rejections and hurts in a desperate effort to reach out for support, acceptance and love from the workers and the group. Some members may engage in nihilistic flight from the group as a way of turning their anger against themselves and showing hostility to members closely bonded to one another.

Larry is a 31-year-old man who overcame physical weakness and disabilities in his childhood, and eventually developed his body to a point of physical perfection that no one in the group could hope to equal. His still admirable physique was perhaps all the more ironic for his having been diagnosed with AIDS a year earlier. Interestingly, when Larry was absent from the group, two members talked at length about how "some gay men are too obsessed with their bodies," but neither mentioned Larry by name, nor did they ever bring up the subject again when he returned. As the weeks went on, Larry's demeanor during sessions changed dramatically over the course of the ninety minutes. He told the group that he always came in "feeling great" and eager to talk about his relationship with his new boyfriend, but that he felt this was too trivial a matter to bring up in a group of people who were as seriously ill as some of these men indeed were. By the end of the meeting he said he would be extremely depressed, and his body language illustrated this as he gradually slumped down in his chair as if he were bearing the cumulative grief of the entire group. With the workers' support (and despite their urging otherwise), Larry eventually decided to take a "leave of absence" from the group because, as he said, he "just couldn't stand being constantly reminded of AIDS." Though he has not returned to the group since he left in February, he does maintain contact with the workers.

Recapitulation

When members acquire a surer realization and acceptance of separation issues in the group, they may reenact past modes of interaction and crises. Active reminiscence about members no longer in the group and the dead occurs frequently.

Stewart, a 35-year-old theatrical executive, returned to the group after a hospitalization for a severely disabling respiratory infection. His physical decline was dramatically evidenced by his recent weight loss of twenty pounds, his grayish pallor and wracking cough. Recently, Stewart had been abandoned by his alcoholic lover and suffered from the discernible stigma of Kaposi's sarcoma lesions on his face, yet he continued to hold a very responsible job which he said gave him "a reason to go on living."

In a quiet, matter-of-fact tone, Stewart said that he would "off" himself when he could no longer work, and that the prospect of returning to his parents in New Haven, should he become more disabled, was "as good as being dead." Larry agreed, indicating that he too had made plans to kill himself "if things get too bad." Other members nodded in agreement, while a few remained quiet and withdrawn. After a period of silence, Stewart expressed sympathy for Rennie, a member who had presumably committed suicide a year earlier. Rennie had expressed deep hurt over being emotionally abandoned by his brother, and disappointment at his inability to remain "in the harness" of daily work. The workers reflected that Stewart and other group members had gone through a great deal of pain and loss recently, and that it was natural to wonder when enough was enough.

The group members then had an elaborated discussion about the importance of preparing "living wills" and medical powers of attorney. The group workers noted that this discussion was very important, since these documents allow people with AIDS to retain control over their lives when they are physically incapacitated.

Suicidal thoughts were natural responses to life-threatening diseases, one worker pointed out, and yet it was painful and difficult for the workers to think of losing any members of the group, since in many ways members' lives were in their hands. If any member decided to take his life, he should not forget to say goodbye to them, in one way or another. Lee, a long-time member, agreed that it was important to be able to say goodbye, and told the group again the tragic suicide of his lover Joe after Joe had been diagnosed with ARC a year and a half earlier. The session ended on a note of palpable sadness.

Flight

The departure of an individual from the group may be impulsive and destructive, or a positive flight characterized by emotional equanimity and the leaving of an enduring legacy to those who remain behind. Positive flight allows for continuity of the group process as departing members feel released from the demands of the group. Group members often undergo a life review process particularly as the prospect of personal mortality becomes apparent. The workers assist members in their life review discussions in the context of the group.

Eighteen months after the group began, the three surviving original members (Lee, Stewart and Jim) became increasingly ill and disabled. Lee came late to a session having missed his subway stop. Embarrassedly, he apologized to a sympathetic group. Lee later related a series of incidents pointing to memory lapses; he noted that there had been a discernible mental change in him, added to Kaposi's sarcoma, cytomegalovirus colitis, tuberculosis, lymphoma and other bodily indignities which he had undergone since his diagnosis two years ago. Group members spoke of becoming demented from HIV infection, and the workers emphasized that as they might discuss physical symptoms, mental ones were also fair game for the group. Lee agreed.

Two sessions later Lee spoke about his worry that Stewart, who was absent from the group, might have KS lesions on his lungs. He was hesitant to discuss this with Stewart in the group. The worker suggested that Stewart could be reached by phone, and might appreciate knowing of Lee's concern. Later, Lee shared a dream-like vision of being in two worlds–this one and a heavenly one. He had a clear image of his beloved mother who died when he was fifteen united with his dead lover and with an old cat that had to be put to sleep because it was too ill to be cared for during his recent hospitalization. He warmly shared memories of his mother and the remote father with whom he could never discuss his being gay. Jim, who had been made totally blind six months earlier by CMV retinitis, and was no longer able to walk, spoke about the abandonment by his fundamentalist Christian parents during his greatest period of need. Yet despite the relentless assaults on his body by AIDS, Jim felt a strange sense of inner strength; he told the group "there's something whole in me that's still untouched by physical illness."

At a subsequent session, Lee talked affectionately about a friend's three-year-old daughter. He told the group that he planned to leave his life insurance to the child for college. Jim announced that he intended to bequeath his personal effects to persons who cared for him over the last few months, particularly his GMHC buddy and his home care worker. "It's pretty obvious how much you love them," one of the workers remarked. Jim nodded in agreement and smiled.

Shortly after this meeting, Lee, Jim and Stewart all became too ill to come to the group, but remained in contact by phone and through home visits by the group workers. The remaining, healthier members had voted to meet on alternate weeks at Jim's home, since he was no longer able to get up or down the three flights of stairs leading to his apartment. But this soon became impossible as Jim became more and more debilitated. Jim said that he appreciated the group's coming to his house, but felt too conspicuous to be seen in this condition. Stewart entered the hospital and died three weeks later, weighing only 90 pounds. Toward the end he was semi-comatose almost constantly, but in a moment of lucidity during the worker's visit to him in the hospital, he asked how Jim and Lee were doing. Jim died four days after Stewart, at home in the arms of a woman friend who was part of a caring team of friends and volunteers that maintained a 24-hour vigil. He left his cat Stanley to Tom, his GMHC buddy.

Lee also became housebound and more disoriented. He was

cared for by a home health team and friends and family. Just prior to Lee's death, his elderly father indicated to friends and the group worker that he had known Lee was gay for 20 years, but did not mention it because as a father he did not want to embarrass his son. Lee heard his father's statement of his acceptance and love for his only son. He glowed with a gentle smile as he talked about his father in the last group session he was able to attend. He died two weeks later. Several of the group, along with the workers, subsequently attended a memorial service for Lee, and his friends made a panel to add to the ever-growing Names Project Memorial Quilt. As he had planned, he left his insurance policy to his friend's three-year-old daughter, and his ballet subscription to his first lover, Sam.

DISCUSSION

The group experience of PWAs represents a multi-level process in which members try to insure their biopsychosocial integrity, while they undergo threats of dissolution of their bodies and their relationships to others. The wish to live fully is challenged by the fear of loss and separation; the group becomes an arena for members to test out solutions that seek to reconcile their unavowed wishes and fears instigated by recognitions of personal vulnerabilities associated with an AIDS diagnosis (Whittaker and Lieberman, 1965). The group workers gently assist group members to explore together the encoded messages associated with loss and separation.

Group workers need to help members focus on finding solutions which avoid the extremes of a morbid, fearful preoccupation with dying and disengagement from life's demands, or a wishful magical scheme to deny the realities of an AIDS diagnosis. Between these two poles lies the safe environment where one can focus on living with AIDS.

In the catalytic atmosphere of group interaction, members develop norms, rituals and an articulated group culture that assists them in facing the vicissitudes of AIDS. The ego strengths of individual members buttressed by the mutual aid process provide a variety of practical, heroic, beneficent and artistic/spiritual solutions to the otherwise unacceptable insults of disease and premature death. The

PWA group experience works best in conjunction with a range of additional crisis services and social supports, to which the worker can help members gain access.

Work with AIDS groups places special demands on group workers, who must gently persevere in exploring with highly vulnerable people what the world might consider painful, taboo subjects of sexuality and death. When others move away from the sick and dying, PWAs may call out for closeness and human touch. Sometimes, despite the most intense efforts, and the most human desire to hold onto life at all costs, group workers must bear witness to tragic loss. The need for support, recognition, and an outlet for cumulative grief responses is a sine qua non for group workers serving people with AIDS. The acknowledgement of our finite powers is never easy. The transformative aspect of this work cannot be overstated. The discovery of the temporal boundaries of existence heightens workers' sense of the moment and the need to instill value into each of those moments.

"How strange a life this first one is," Charles Ludlam wrote in his unique version of *Camille* (1987). Strange and wonderful, and worth every minute. This is the lesson that group work with people with AIDS teaches us all.

REFERENCES

Buber, M. 1970. *I and Thou.* New York: Charles Scribner's Sons.

Gambe, R. and Getzel, G.S. 1988. "Group Work with Gay Men with AIDS," *Social Casework* (in press).

Garland, J.A., Jones, H.E. and Kolodny, R.L. 1965. "A Model for Stages of Development in Social Work Groups," in S. Bernstein, ed. *Explorations in Group Work.* Boston: Boston University Press.

Getzel, G.S. 1987. *Overview of the Psychosocial Issues Concerning AIDS.* New York: Gay Men's Health Crisis Publications.

Heap, K. 1977. *Group Theory for Social Workers.* Oxford: Pergamon Press.

Lopez, D. and Getzel, G.S. 1984. "Helping Gay AIDS Patients in Crisis," *Social Casework,* (September).

Lopez, D. and Getzel, G.S. 1987. "Survival Strategies for Volunteers Working with Persons with AIDS," *Social Casework,* (January).

Ludlam, C. 1987. *The Collected Plays of Charles Ludlam.* New York: Grove Press.

Northen, H. 1988. *Social Work with Groups*, 2nd ed. New York: Columbia University Press.

Saroyan, W. 1959. *The Time of Your Life*, in *Famous American Plays of the 1930s*. New York: Laurel Press.

Walker, G. 1988. "Confronting the Specter of AIDS," *The Family Therapy Networker*, (January/February).

Whittaker, D. and Lieberman, M.A. 1965. *Psychotherapy Through the Group Process*. New York: Aldine Press.

Yalom, I. 1985. *Theory and Practice of Group Psychotherapy*, 3rd ed. New York: Basis Books.

An AIDS Bereavement Support Group: One Model of Intervention in a Time of Crisis

Robert C. Amelio

INTRODUCTION

In February 1987 an AIDS bereavement support group began under the auspices of the AIDS Action Committee of Massachusetts. The purpose of this group is to offer bereaved individuals who have lost someone to AIDS an opportunity to mourn the death with others suffering similar losses. The AIDS Action Committee (AAC) is the major provider of services for people affected by AIDS in New England. This group is one of more than a dozen support groups offered through the AAC. At the time this group began it was the only bereavement group offered with membership open to both straight and gay, men and women, lovers, widows, adult children, friends, siblings, parents–essentially anyone who lost someone to AIDS. This paper will focus on several aspects of this particular group including demographics and group structure, AIDS bereavement issues, countertransference issues, and advantages and disadvantages of the group model.

AIDS BEREAVEMENT

The bereavement of a loved one is a difficult period in an individual's life, one that can last an indeterminate amount of time. The death of a loved one to AIDS may complicate this process of grieving due to the stigma associated with this disease. Worden (1982) listed three conditions that may complicate the grieving process: (1) when the loss is socially unspeakable; (2) when the loss is socially negated; (3) in the absence of a social support network. AIDS bereavement may and often does carry all of these conditions with it leaving bereaved individuals more vulnerable to complications in their grieving, the potential resolution of their grief, and the reconstruction of their lives.

There are many examples of how society stigmatizes people with AIDS (PWAs) and their survivors. Some forms of this stigmatization take shape in ostracism and isolation by family, friends, and community (Batchelor, 1984; Geis, Fuller & Rush, 1988; Morin, 1984), loss of jobs (Baker, 1988; Kaplan, 1988), loss of housing (Baker, 1988; Kaplan, 1988), and even a house-burning (Monmaney, 1987).

The response of PWAs and their survivors to this stigma varies. Some responses are: the decision to keep the true nature of the disease a secret (Kaplan, 1988; Oerlemans-Bunn, 1988; Walker, 1987), isolating self from others (Geis et al., 1988; Oerlemans-Bunn, 1988), fearing intimate contact with others (Morin, Charles, Malyon, 1984), and not grieving publicly (Kaplan, 1988).

Many of the bereavement issues of the survivors relate directly to their feelings about the stigmatization they have experienced while their loved one was still living with AIDS. These include issues of: anger at society, fear of rejection in new relationships, suicidal thoughts, self-punishing thoughts, severe depression, fear of developing new relationships, fear of being HIV (human immunodeficiency virus) positive, curtailed sexual activity, thoughts of being a leper, and keeping the true cause of a loved one's death to AIDS a secret (Batchelor, 1984; Geis et al., 1988; Kaplan, 1988; Monmaney, 1987; Morin, 1984; Morin et al., 1984; Oerlemans-Bunn, 1988; Walker, 1987; Whitmore, 1988).

GROUP STRUCTURE

As a result of the perceived stigma of bereaved individuals who have lost someone to AIDS this particular bereavement group was formed with three basic goals: (1) to provide a forum for bereaved individuals to discuss their feelings and other issues related to the deaths; (2) to create a mutual-aid network for group members; (3) to enable and empower members to deal with their grief reactions and the stigma and isolation often experienced due to AIDS.

The group meets every other week for 1 1/2 hours in the greater Boston area. All members are screened by telephone contact by the AAC group program coordinator who then refers the individual to one of the two group co-leaders. We ask each member for a three session commitment after which the individual can decide when to terminate from the group. The average length of stay is 4-5 months though many members have continued with the group for 6 months or more. Since the group began in 1987 more than 30 individuals have come to the group.

Co-led by a gay male social work graduate student and a straight female psychologist, the group has welcomed inclusion of any person who has lost someone to AIDS. Our first members were a gay man who lost several friends, a straight woman whose fiancee died of AIDS, and a straight woman whose 38-year-old daughter died. Members join at various stages of their bereavement. Some have come to the group two weeks after the death, others months or years later.

Each group meeting begins with a photograph exchange in which members pass around any pictures of the deceased. This procedure was initiated by the members themselves who spontaneously began to bring in pictures and other mementos and thus a formal period was created so that anyone has the opportunity to share photographs or other articles. After the photo session each member "checks in." A rule of the group is that check-in includes the name of the person who died of AIDS and when that person died. Any other information a member wishes to bring up about the weeks since the last meeting or the grieving process is also welcome at this time. Once all members have checked-in (with the option to pass) discussion is open to any issues the members want to discuss. Any member present for the first time to the group is allowed more time during the check-in to talk in detail about the illness and death of the loved one and the subsequent bereavement.

For many who have come to the group it has been the only place they have been able to talk about and mourn their losses in a supportive and non-judgmental atmosphere. The mutual aid network that has developed within the group had been a primary reason for its successful continuation. Members exchange addresses and phone numbers, have visited each other during hospitalizations, and socialize together. The members are extremely committed to attend each meeting. One member attended the day after being released from the hospital for lung surgery. The actual illnesses, AIDS-related or not, of the members raise great concern for the other members. When a member has missed a meeting and is known to be ill several members will call him and offer any help they can provide. Perhaps this is their way of helping yet another person cope with illness, another way of being a caregiver, which for most is a familiar role. Perhaps it is also their fear of losing someone else to AIDS that compels them to be especially sensitive to one another.

The backgrounds, professionally and personally, of the two co-leaders have also influenced the continuation of this group. Having a straight female psychologist and a gay male social worker lead the group represents an inclusive atmosphere and has enabled both men and women, straight and gay, to be comfortable in the group. Though no one has asked us about our individual sexual orientations I believe the physical presence of a man and a woman encourages all members to feel welcome.

GROUP ISSUES

Bereavement of the death of a loved one to AIDS has similarities and differences with bereavement by other forms of death. A bereaved individual usually learns there is a societally-imposed time limit in which grieving is supposed to occur. After this time limit other people begin to wonder when the bereaved person will "snap out of it." A grieving person finds other people are not comfortable talking about death or how much the deceased is missed and thus tends to suppress his other true feelings from others often during bereavement (which may last only a few months for some but years for others). The bereaved individual might wear the clothes of the deceased, sleep on the deceased's side of the bed, or be forgetful and view these and other such behaviors as bizarre. Feelings of sadness, anger, anxiety, relief, fatigue, or helplessness might overtake the bereaved at unexpected and sudden times and seem overwhelming. These are some of the experiences reported by many of the group members and abound in literature about grief which survivors of losses from AIDS as well as other deaths seem to have in common.

Bereavement of a death to AIDS, which is seen by many in our society as a stigmatizing disease, has its own set of issues that may complicate the grieving and reconstruction process. These issues form the core of the work of this group and have been experienced to some degree by all of the members of the group. The major AIDS-related issues presented in this paper are: (1) feeling stigmatized; (2) feeling isolated; (3) asking the questions: "will I be next to get AIDS?"; "should I be tested for HIV?"; "who gave it to whom?" (4) the difficulty in being able to grieve publicly; (5) cumulative losses to AIDS; (6) AIDS overload.

Stigma and Isolation

The issues of stigma and isolation are the most commonly presented concerns in the group, particularly for newer members. These seem equally relevant to gay as well as straight members. One member, a woman whose 38-year-old daughter died of AIDS told us:

> No one besides my husband knows how Susan died. If my friends knew she had AIDS it would soil her memory, they'll look down on her, it would take away any respect anyone had for her. I'll never tell anyone what killed her.

Another member, a gay man has said:

> Being gay, I thought all of our friends would support us and help us out. It was as if we had done something bad, something

wrong. After Joe died they were all there at the funeral but only a few have bothered to contact me since then.

A woman whose boyfriend died of AIDS said:

Max had gone clean (from intravenous drug use) 2 years before he died. He was an example to his other (drug-using) friends of someone who was making it. And then–wham!–he gets AIDS and is dead in two weeks. And not one of our friends was there to help us out. Suddenly we were both untouchable. I think it was too scary for them. If Max had gone clean and got AIDS what was going to happen to them?

This stigma may remain with the survivor as he begins to explore new romantic relationships. One man told the group:

I want to date again but what do I say–oh, by the way, my lover died of AIDS, but don't worry, I'm o.k.? I'm negative now but who knows what's in my system. I feel like a leper.

Our decision to open the group to anyone who has lost someone to AIDS, not only gay men, or parents, or family members, was based in part on our desire to de-stigmatize the disease and create a group of individuals from all walks of life who shared the common bond of losing someone to AIDS. By encouraging parents, wives, gay and straight lovers, adult children, and siblings to talk about their grief with one another the concept of AIDS as a "gay disease" has dissipated and the isolation experienced by so many of the members in their lives outside of the group is diminished.

Unanswerable Questions

For many of the members in the group their bereavement is complicated by unanswerable questions. A primary question members ask is: "Will I be next?" This is particularly true of the bereaved romantic partners in the group, though others have asked this question. Other concerns are whether or not to be tested for exposure to HIV and wondering who gave the disease to whom.

Some discussion about these questions has been:

> I've been tested positive and now I'm just waiting. I know I'll get it at some point. And knowing doesn't really help.

> I don't know if I'm positive or negative. I'm never going to be with someone again so what difference does it make?

> I just live with the assumption that I am positive and live every day as fully as I can.

> I want to know but I'm afraid. I would only worry more than I already do now.

Though no one can provide any satisfactory answers to these questions it seems once the members verbalize their concerns and are allowed to talk about them at length they are able to ease some anxiety and focus on other bereavement issues as well. Unfortunately, AIDS is a disease characterized by many questions and not enough answers. Survivors carry the burden of these questions long after the loved one has died.

Public Mourning

Some members have expressed their difficulty in mourning publicly for the deceased which is another condition that may complicate the grieving process. Some of the gay men in the group who are not "out" at work have had problems explaining to their bosses and co-workers the true relationship to their "friend" who has died. For some of the straight members in the group it has been equally as difficult to mourn publicly. Some have feared the reactions of friends, co-workers, and relatives to their news that someone close to them has died of AIDS thus forcing them to hide the true cause of death or to withdraw from these people at a time when support and comfort are so important. One member, a public school teacher who lost her husband of over 20 years to AIDS has chosen not to tell most of her co-workers how he died because of her fear of the perceived or real repercussions in doing so. Having to hide the truth of the disease, or even more extreme, that someone very close to the member has died has caused guilt and prolonged grief for some of the members. For many the group is the only place they have to speak honestly about their loss without fear of judgement.

Cumulative AIDS Losses

The issue of cumulative, compounded losses is of particular importance to some of the gay men in the group. One man has lost six close friends in the last year. Almost every member knows someone else who has died of AIDS, has tested positive, or has ARC (AIDS related condition). One member was faced with the news in a short period of time that his two ex-lovers both had AIDS. It is as if these members have no rest from grief. Their grieving becomes chronic. As soon as they feel ready to face the world again another death occurs in their lives.

AIDS Overload

Another closely related issue is one of AIDS overload, that is, being surrounded by AIDS. Members have spoken about their inability to escape the reality of AIDS for even a short time due to the proliferation of articles in the media on AIDS, television programs on AIDS, conferences and seminars on AIDS, AIDS memorial services, AIDS-fund raising events. While they acknowledge the importance of this saturation to raise public consciousness to the magnitude of this disease, many members express anger at being reminded constantly of AIDS and thus the death of the loved one they now mourn. One woman poignantly said: "Seeing AIDS everywhere I go reminds me every day of my own pain. Just for one day I would like not to have a public reminder of my husband's death, of the intense pain I am living with." For some members the daily reality of AIDS becomes even more personal when tested positive or at the onset of symptoms of ARC. One such man said: "Everywhere I look there are reminders about AIDS. And now, just when I was getting used to them, I test positive, I start getting a bad cough and there it is right in my face every day again."

The group has been an outlet for all members to express their fears, mourn their losses, and share their rage. Through mutual support and non-evaluative listening these issues can seem less overwhelming and isolating.

COUNTERTRANSFERENCE ISSUES

There are several issues I have had to examine for myself as a co-leader of this group. The fact that the majority of members have been gay men has caused me to come face-to-face with my own anxiety about AIDS in my life and that of my lover. When I first began leading the group there were moments in which I felt helpless to intervene because I was so suddenly immersed in my own thoughts of mortality as I listened to the members' stories. I have often found myself thinking about the question: "Will I too be next?" At times when a member tells about the special shared moments he misses with his partner I think about the special relationship I have with my lover and the void that would be left in my life if he were to die. During and after group meetings I often recount my own losses which rekindles feelings of sadness. There have been moments in the group when my own thoughts about these losses have pulled me away from the work of the group and I have to focus even more on what the members are saying. I too sometimes feel overloaded by AIDS and feel a sense of compounded losses through these peoples' experiences. When a new member comes to a group meeting for the first time I have to struggle with my own resistance toward the person, not wanting to listen to yet another story of pain.

I have been able to discuss these thoughts and feelings openly with my co-leader which has enabled me to continue with this work. The leaders of the other AAC support groups also meet in monthly supervision which allows us the opportunity to hear these issues raised and discussed in depth.

When I first began leading the group, because it was my first experience leading a group, I could not imagine coming back week after week to have these feelings and issues surface within me. Now I understand they have been part of my process of coping with AIDS and loss. I believe this has allowed me to develop a more enriched empathy with the members of the group and has increased my ability to be present, intervene, and create a safe environment for the members.

ADVANTAGES AND DISADVANTAGES
OF GROUP MODEL

As with any group model there are advantages and disadvantages to the structure we have chosen for this group. An open-ended group such as this has a disadvantage in comparison with a time-limited group in that new members can come into the group at any time and at various stages of group development. Though each member seems to have become fully incorporated into the group there is a period of "catching up" which new members go through to learn the personal histories of each person concerning their loss to AIDS and to become acquainted with the group culture.

New members are generally at a different, earlier stage of grieving than older members, which can be both helpful and difficult for the group. When a new member talks about the initial pain and anguish over the loss of a loved one or is confused about unexplained behaviors such as forgetfulness, the older members can reassure the new person that this struggle is normal and one that they too have experienced. Older members can relate their own strategies for how they handled the painful initial period after the death and the coping mechanisms that worked best for them. This information often seems more authentic to the new member coming from someone in the group rather than from a friend or mental health professional who has not suffered a similar loss. In this respect older members become teachers as well as peers to the new members and are able to experience a sense of generativity toward the new members. This also creates a cycle of support from a more "experienced" member to a newcomer which eases the inclusion of the new person into the group.

There have been times when a new member has brought up what is an old issue in the group, but new to this member, which requires the group to go back to that emotional experience. This can be even more painful than the first telling of the event. As one member said: "Doug died once but I live through his death 1000 times." However, this retelling of an already told story can have a more dramatic healing effect than the first telling. We have found that the same details, feelings, or events cannot be told enough by some members. This is a way to heal themselves of their grief, and a way of making the death more real to them.

Though it has not become one yet, the lack of a personal, face-to-face interview could be a problem. Some bereaved individuals may need more than the services of this support group to support them during this period and may need more intensive therapeutic work. We would have no way of knowing this until that person was in the group. A personal interview could also help a prospective member decide if the group seemed appropriate to serve that person's needs.

The open-ended commitment asked of each member allows the individual to personally decide when to terminate from the group. This can be a very empowering decision. Though every person leaves for unique reasons there is a sense of growth and change which marks a person's leaving. We welcome members to come back to the group at any time, though no one has done this yet.

One of the most positive characteristics of this group model is its make-up: gay, straight, lovers, wives, adult children, siblings, parents, and friends. This inclusiveness has decreased the isolation of the members and the categorization of "who gets AIDS and who doesn't."

A bereavement support group for people who have lost someone to AIDS is a powerful testament to the importance of support and mutual aid to these individuals. This paper has highlighted several key factors to consider in working with AIDS bereaved individuals. These factors include the relevant issues in working with this population, group structure, the pros and cons of this particular group model, and possible countertransference issues for group leaders or individual therapists to consider.

AIDS will continue to claim lives for years to come. Through my experience in co-leading this group and sitting with the members' pain, tears, laughter, and hope, I can attest to its usefulness as a means of intervention. It is unfortunate to say that many more of these groups are needed now and will be needed into the future. The social work tradition of group work for people in need is a natural avenue for social workers to reach out and make a difference during this time of crisis.

REFERENCES

Baker, J.N. (1988, April 4). Needing a place to die. *Newsweek*, 24-25.

Batchelor, W. (1984). AIDS: A public health and psychological emergency. *American Psychologist*, 39 (11), 1279-1284.

Geis, S.B., Fuller, R.L., & Rush, J. (1986). Lovers of AIDS victims: psychosocial stresses and counseling needs. *Death Studies*, 10 (1), 43-53.

Kaplan, L. (1988, January/February). Guilt and AIDS. *The Family Therapy NETWORKER*, 40-41, 80.

Monmaney, T. (1987, September 7). Kids with AIDS. *Newsweek*, 51-59.

Morin, S.F. (1984). AIDS in one city. *American Psychologist*, 39 (11), 1294-1296.

Morin, S.F., Charles, K.A., & Maylon, A.K. (1984). The psychological impact of AIDS on gay men. *American Psychologist*, 39 (11), 1288-1293.

Oerlemans-Bunn, M. (1988, April). On being gay, single, and bereaved. *American Journal of Nursing*, 472-476.

Walker, L.A. (1987, June 21). What comforts AIDS families. *The New York Times Magazine*, 16-23.

Whitmore, G. (1988, January 31). Bearing witness. *The New York Times Magazine*, 15-16, 49-54.

Worden, J.W. (1982). *Grief Counseling and Grief Therapy*. New York: Springer Publishing Co.

Social Work Practice with Groups in the Church Context: A Family Life Ministry Model in an Inner-City Church

Patricia Lawson Bailey

THE CHURCH AS A CONTEXT FOR PRACTICE

Church members come together around a common belief system. The large mega-churches with several thousand members operate as formal bureaucratic systems, but most churches are small voluntary organizations. Some denominations have more hierarchy than others, but even these operate daily parish ministry with informal structures. Churches depend on the favor of the membership, and tradition determines agenda more than present environment. Instead of a formal structure that provides consistent processes, the typical church operates as an informal system. This informality provides uneven decision making that is often unique and unpredictable. The social worker must watch and listen for distinctive qualities and values of the client system without passing judgment on them. Projecting results and planning interventions with this client system may be elusive and unpredictable (Garland, 1988; Garland, Rainbow, & Bailey, 1988). It is easy to forget social work values and deny self-determination with such a difficult client system.

The unique environment of the church calls for a skilled social worker. While helping and caring have been a central focus of the church for thousands of years, ministry practice has not usually been professionalized. However, social work processes fit comfortably with the nature of congregational life, so that large numbers of

55

social workers elect the church as a context for practice. Social work as a profession can little afford to ignore this mediating structure that has the trust of so many.

THE COMMUNITY AND BAPTIST TABERNACLE

Baptist Tabernacle is a 90-year-old church in Portland, a community located in west Louisville, Kentucky. In the 1950s, this congregation was a thriving church with 500 persons in attendance each week. During the 1960s, dozens of families fled the community as integration became a growing concern. When riots stormed that section of the city, out-migration from the community continued even more heavily.

By 1980, 14,248 people remained in the Portland area, the majority of whom were low-income Whites; Blacks composed only 7 percent of the population (Census of Population and Housing, 1980). While only one Black family participates in the church membership, the membership policy of the church is inclusive. All family life ministries are open to Black persons, and they do receive emergency assistance. It is unlikely that Black persons will become active in the congregation, however, because there are two Black Baptist churches in the community.

In 1980, the national average for household annual income in the U.S. was $20,306, compared to the average for Portland households of $11,339. Twenty-seven percent of Portland families live below the poverty level compared to the national average of 9.5 percent. Women head 46 percent of low income families in Portland (Census of Population, 1980).

Many Portland residents have been unsuccessful in school. Fifty-two percent of persons 16-19 years old are high school dropouts. Forty-two percent of persons 25 and older have a grade school education or less (Census of Population, 1980).

Teenagers and children in this neighborhood struggle for survival along with crime, unemployment, and lack of parental supervision. Teen pregnancy is also a growing problem for many youngsters, and lifelong changes occur because of teenage pregnancy. When a teen does not finish school, unemployment will follow and the probability of long-term poverty increases (Davis, 1988).

As Portland's population declined, so did the membership of Baptist Tabernacle. While some of the Tabernacle families drove back to their church, many moved to suburban congregations. The church members remaining from the community, for the most part, are aged or have special needs. Many of the members in the congregation have reached a majority age, and over 750 members have died in the last 26 years. These factors have contributed to declining resources and heightened needs as the congregation struggles for life.

The decline of Baptist Tabernacle is a reflection of the community at large. As middle income families moved out of the community, housing turned to rental property, and absentee slum lords seldom kept housing repaired. Arson and dilapidated housing are signs of the hopelessness of many residents. Many single parents live in the community and are teenage mothers. Also many aged residents live on fixed incomes. High unemployment reflects the high number of school dropouts, and poverty determines the low quality of life as citizens strive to provide basic needs for themselves and their families.

Traditional church programming proved unsuccessful in meeting the needs of the community as well as the church family. In 1985, the congregation hired a part-time church social worker to design and implement a Family Life Ministry. Along with the pastor and church leadership, she designed a family life program that would be acceptable to the membership who did not live in the community and that would reach community residents as well.

Tabernacle became a field placement setting for the Carver School of Church Social Work. First and second year MSW students practice 10 and 20 hours respectively each week and students read Hartford's *Groups in Social Work* as the theoretical base for social group work practice. Students from the program directing (administration and management) concentration and the FIG concentration (direct practice with Families, Individuals, and Groups) have practiced at Tabernacle now for three years.

FAMILY LIFE MINISTRY AND SOCIAL WORK WITH GROUPS

With little or no money and few supporters, the church social worker designed the Family Life Ministry around social work with groups. "The naturalness of group process and the nonsynthetic qualities of the activities of the group predetermine that the professional posture shall be warm, informal, and free of remote authoritarianism" (Papell & Rothman, 1966, p. 11). The group format also offers a sense of community that is advantageous to individual crisis intervention models (Sarason, 1974).

Social work practice with groups fits well with the informal voluntary nature of congregational life, and several groups were already ongoing part of Tabernacle life. It was important to keep change to a minimum to prevent reaction rather than proaction. Consequently, the Family Life Ministry needed to be structured into the organization so institutionalization would come as the months and years passed. The program design included four categories of social work practice: (1) group work, (2) family assistance, (3) community concerns, and (4) special projects. Representatives from each of the social work practice areas were added to the church council to coordinate with other church functions. The congregation designated 4.3% of the weekly offerings for the Family Life Ministry.

Activity Groups and Support Groups
with Senior Adults

The Senior Swingers are senior adults who have been meeting weekly for more than a dozen years at Tabernacle. Some Swingers are church members and some are community friends. Activities such as field trips and crafts have been a focus of the group. Educational programs on topics such as nutrition and health add variety to their calendar, and the swingers share a pot-luck dinner monthly. Birthday parties and holiday parties highlight special celebrations. The Swingers are getting older and new younger members are not coming into the group.

Social work practice with the Swingers is moving more in the direction of support groups for widows and reminiscing groups. During these last years, it would be easy for these persons to become isolated. Club groups in trusted institutions like the church can assist the elderly with social and financial functions (Abrahams, 1972). Social work practice with this coveted group takes priority over other new groups at Baptist Tabernacle.

In a sense, the group for the aged is the way the church deals with its "social responsibility" (Papell & Rothman, 1966). Swingers have provided "intellectual and social enhancement" (Hartford, 1976), as well as a mutual aid system. The group has aided the aged in the congregation to "strengthen and develop social networks" (Abels & Abels, 1980).

The support and care for one another binds the group together (Gottlieb). Natural helping is the emphasis as members transport each other to doctor's appointments and shopping, telephone each other regularly, and visit in the homes of those who are ill and/or homebound (Silverman, 1980).

Case management around individual needs of the aged has led to brokering with community agencies in support of Swingers. Cases have included working with social security officials, adult protective services, long term care facilities, hospitals, medicare officials, and the housing authority. As the Swingers become frail elderly, they will require more case management with individuals and families.

Self-Help Groups for Chemically Dependent Persons

The other group that existed before the program design was the Saturday night Alcoholics Anonymous group. Some 35 community persons meet at the church each week to participate in AA. Recently an Alanon group started and an activities group for the children of AA, and Alanon serves some 12 to 15 children.

Social work professionals are learning that existing social networks can expand to self-help groups. Too often the professional role has been to analyze the person rather than allow the natural relationships to emerge into a group. The AA group that meets at Tabernacle comes from the neighborhood. New members and persons who "slip" are welcome. The church social workers have learned more from the AA group than any gain the group has experienced because of the workers.

The staff has taken 16 hours of Core Skills with COPES (Council on the Prevention and Education of Substances) and 12 hours of training on working with youth. This area of social work practice will expand as recovering volunteers become involved. The leadership vision for this area of social work practice includes family practice with chemically dependent families.

Self-Help for Women

The process of self-help is based on the following assumptions:

- Each person makes appropriate use of the resources as he or she can; each person is his or her own authority about what he/she needs.
- All of us know more than any one of us.
- Openness and honesty are important (Mallory, 1984).

Self-help describes a "broad variety of helping activities that may represent a continuum of arrangements for engaging in mutual aid" (Pancoast, Parker & Froland, 1983).

In 1985, a self-help group began for women when two women presented a need to the church social worker and requested that the group start. The women group members called themselves the "I Will Survive Group." Members of the group were rape victims, spouse abuse victims, divorcing persons, and single parents. These 8-10 women made wooden ducks and sold them to generate money for activities. The group skated, picnicked, and took field trips. They worked on self-esteem issues, parenting, coping, finances, etc. Two of the women entered college, one got full-time employment for the first time, and the battered woman moved into the spouse abuse shelter while child custody was fought in the courts.

The women helped each other by calling, being together, sharing their stories and their coping skills. When monies were short, they pooled their knowledge about welfare benefits and how to use the system. When court dates came, a friend from the group went along. None of these women were church members and community people saw the church as a service delivery agency.

The social worker, as facilitator prepared a gambit or exercise for starting the group (NiCarthy, Meriam, & Coffman, 1984; Dossick & Shea, 1988; Eberhardt, 1978). Group members became actively involved immediately. Members often brought a problem to the group when crisis overcame their thinking and living. "Put very simply, people depend(ed) upon others for survival needs and improved quality of life" (Wasserman & Danforth, 1988). The members supported, showed care, and shared coping devices with each other as the group bonded together.

Case management and family assistance came out of the group experience. The Family Life Ministry of the church maintained a food pantry, clothes store, and financial assistance. The church social worker negotiated with child protective services, treatment centers for the chemically dependent, food banks, and schools as the women requested further support from the family life ministry of the church.

The social worker's role in the group was coordinator, enabler, facilitator and catalyst. To facilitate means to make easier, to guide, and to lead. Leadership in the group moved from member to member according to the discussion (Mallory, 1984). Volunteers from the congregation led activities for the children during group time. One group member acted as the lead volunteer and telephoned and arranged for transportation each week. Group members chose topics from assessment lists and planned together. The social worker failed to set up an evaluation pretest and posttest, but client feedback showed the group to be successful in meeting the needs of group members. The group met for 12 months and ended as contracted.

Self-Help for Single Parents

Two of the women from the "I Will Survive" group started a group for Single Parents the following Fall semester after being out of group during the summer. The Single Parent's Self-Help group gathered with a church social worker and planned for the group. The social worker began making home visits to insure the success of the group (Kurland, 1978). The group phases and theory base followed Hartford's *Groups in Social Work.*

The professional was coordinator, enabler, and facilitator. The social worker prepared exercises for the group as back up, but always hoped for group members to take responsibility for the group. Sometimes they did and sometimes they did not. The church social worker coordinated child care, refreshments, and transportation. The church social worker prepared a Procedural Manual so the next social worker would not have to re-invent the process. Also the Manual was made available to other churches at a small cost through *Models for Ministry,* Volume III. The hope is that social work practice with single parents will become a popular church intervention.

By the end of the semester, group members completed a posttest to determine knowledge or skills gained around the selected topics. Single-system design was used to evaluate the success of particular interventions. Client feedback was also positive (Davis, 1988).

Case management with individuals and family members followed as requested. The social worker served as broker with various human service agencies to meet client needs. Case conferences proved appropriate when multiple professionals from various agencies worked with the same client. Practice often revolved around the children of the Single Parent. The Single Parent group is still meeting, though the facilitator and some of its members have changed.

Special Needs Groups

Two short-term groups to serve special needs validated the church social worker and helped middle-class church members identify with the Family Life Ministry. A Saturday morning Stress Management Group met in the home of a church leader. Neighbors and friends came for 8 weeks and the group celebrated with a family picnic on the 9th week. While client feedback was positive, different people attended each week and the group never reached a stage of self-maintenance (Hartford, 1971). The group did meet educational needs. It was exciting to see the church in the neighborhood with neighbors relying on each other for mutual aid in everyday exchanges (Froland, Pancoast, Chapman & Kimboko, 1981).

The second special needs group dealt with grief. Church members who lost parents and spouses came for six Sunday nights. The social worker's role in these meetings was expert and facilitator. Church leadership attended these group sessions and the church social worker gained needed credibility in the congregation.

TOPS (Take Off Pounds Sensibly) is three years old. It began when a church member volunteered to start this self-help group based on her own personal need. Her doctor told her there was no weight loss group in Portland. The self-help group meets on Thursday evenings and attendance ranges from 8 to 12. The church bought the professional scale for the group and the church social worker checks regularly with the group members for evaluation.

A community resident telephoned the church social worker to inquire about having a Tough Love Group. This self-help group assists parents in setting limits with children and youth. After the woman presented her need to the church council, the congregation approved this new group as a part of the Family Life Ministry. Four to six members meet weekly to help each other set limits and not rescue their children from the consequences of their decisions. This new self-help group is popular already in its early months.

Self-Help for Youth

Two years ago, social work practice with youth began with Rebound. Rebound began as a camp experience when the youth planned a tent camping week. Upon returning home from camp, the youth decided to keep Rebound and make it a teen club. The stated goal for Rebound was "to bridge the gap between the community and church" (Day, 1987). The youth needed a safe place to hang out, some positive role models, and the opportunity to talk honestly about issues that concerned them (Day, 1987:76).

The church social worker planned with the youth council to have a Saturday night Rebound program which would include recreation (ping pong, billiards, and table games), and a small group time called Straight Talk. The Straight Talk group gave youth an opportunity to talk about sex, drugs, parents, and school problems. This Saturday night small group changed the second year.

The second year of Straight Talk developed into a peer counseling group (Vorrath & Brendtro, 1985) with the curriculum materials based on interviewing skills (Middleman & Goldberg, 1974). The peer counseling need emerged from an assessment survey. The survey results said that these teens would not go to a human service agency if they had a problem (Day, 1987). After training, the peer counselors served in their schools.

The group context was also selected for supervision and training for the peer counselors, using role playing techniques, participative techniques, and peer supervision (Parry, 1979). The group ended when the church social worker, a social work student, graduated in May, 1988.

Mutual Help Group for Teen Moms

In the Spring of 1988, one of the church social workers started a teen mothers mutual aid support group after school at the local high school. A community needs assessment had identified five significant social problems. One of these was teen pregnancy. Baptist Tabernacle voted as a congregation to focus on the problem of teen pregnancy and authorized one of the church social workers to plan an appropriate intervention.

A teen mother in the congregation was interviewed about her interest in beginning a mutual aid group. She responded positively and brought a couple of other teen moms with her to the group. Natural relationships emerged into helping networks. This intervention helped the teen moms understand that others shared their circumstances, the "all-in-the-same-boat phenomenon" (Wasserman & Danforth, 1988:141; Silverman, 1980).

This client group would not respond to an expert leader as well as they responded to each other. There was less concern with the group members' past than with their present commonality of experience (Silverman, 1980:40). "The small group can provide an invaluable opportunity for mutual aid, mutual problem solving and positive growth for adolescents" (Gitterman & Shulman, 1986:125).

The church social worker arranged for space, child care, and transportation and did outreach for group members. The professional role was to meet with the group, control the resources, and direct the flow of the meeting (Trabue, 1988). The leader set the tone for the group with a philosophy of acceptance.

The group members chose weekly topics, group goals and rules. The goals revolved around coping skills and self-esteem issues. The social worker designed evaluation tools for the group. Single-system design, pre- and post-tests and client feedback assisted the social worker in determining the success of the intervention.

Midway into the group experience, the school dismissed three of the group members because they lived in another school district. The group never recovered from the loss of the three members and struggled to survive until the end of the semester.

In addition to these support groups, the church social workers have planned a Family Life Festival each May for three years. Church members identified choices from an assessment list. Groups were offered for each age group. The following groups were among the offerings these past three years:

1. Child Lures–Teach the Children to Say No
2. Hunger in Our Community
3. Retirement Preparation
4. Caring for Aging Parents
5. Caring for Families in Crisis
6. Sex Education
7. Wellness/Stress Management
8. Parenting
9. Mid-life Crisis
10. Marriage Enrichment
11. Stepfamilies
12. Say No to Drugs

The purpose of the Festival is to educate and do consciousness-raising in the congregation. Attendance has been strong and the public relations and marketing to the church family has strengthened support for social work practice in the church. Evaluations last year indicated that the congregation wanted a Fall Festival as well as the May Festival. While this special practice is time consuming and drains an already overworked staff, the results make the effort worthwhile. It is hard to believe that the same congregation that was so resistant three years ago is requesting additional exposure to social issues.

CONCLUSIONS

As is often the case, hindsight provides more understanding than future planning. Social work practice with groups matches the church context. The strongest groups at Baptist Tabernacle have resulted from natural relationships that formed helping networks. Friends brought friends to their group meetings. These natural helping networks then expanded as the relationships came together in the group.

Leadership is tricky for self-help and mutual aid. The leader must direct conversations and not act as expert. Group members must share responsibilities and planning. The Tough Love and TOPS groups have not had a social worker. They seem to be strong and stable. The group members take responsibility more readily. However, the groups with church social workers for leaders use assessment interventions, features which the groups started by community persons do not have. Regardless of this difference, the most important ingredient in family life groups in the Tabernacle context has to do with creating a group environment that is warm, informal, safe, and nurturing for its members. The value of a nurturing group climate should not be surprising news for caregivers. Over and over the words ring in the caregivers' ears: affirm, encourage, support, collaborate, and negotiate! Basic helping, whether in group or not, is about RELATIONSHIP (Perlman, 1979). The group is one way of bringing people together. This warm, supportive kind of community also describes the best of what is known as the "church."

REFERENCES

Abels, S. & Abels, P. (1980). Social group work's contextual purposes. *Social Work with Groups*, 3 (3), 25-37.

Abrams, P. (1980). Social change, social networks and neighborhood care, *Social Work Services*, 22, 12-23.

Davis, Angela D. (1988). A procedure manual for a self-help group for single mothers, *Models For Ministry*. Vol. III, Louisville, KY: Paul R. Adkins Institute for Research and Training in Church Social Work.

Day, Robert (1987). Rebound: A model for inner-city youth ministry, *Models For Ministry*, Vol. II, Louisville, KY: Paul R. Adkins Institute for Research and Training in Church Social Work.

Dossick, J. & Shea, E. (1988). *Creative therapy: 52 exercises for groups*. Sarasota, Florida: Professional Resource Exchange.

Eberhardt, Louise Yolton (1987). *Working with women's groups*, Vol. I & 2. Duluth, MN: Whole Person Press.

Froland et al. (1981). *Helping networks and human services.* Beverly Hills: Sage Publishers.

Garland, D. (1988). The church as a context for social work practice, *Review & Expositor*, 85 (2), 255-266.

Garland, D., Rainbow, J. & Bailey, P. (1988). *Working with churches.* Unpublished manuscript.

Gitterman, A. & Shulman, L. (1986). *Mutual aid groups and the life cycle.* Itasca, Il; F.E. Peacock, Publishers.

Gottlieb, B.H. (1983). *Social support strategies: guidelines for mental health practice.* Beverly Hills, CA: Sage Publishers.

Hamlin, E. & Timberlake, E. (1982). Peer group supervision for supervisors, *Social Casework*, 63 (2), 82-87.

Hartford, Margaret E. (1971). *Groups in Social Work*, New York: Columbia University Press.

Kurland, R. (1978). Planning: The neglected component of group development. *Social Work with Groups*, 1 (20), 173-178.

Mallory, Lucretia (1984). *Leading self-help Groups.* New York: Family Services of America.

Middleman, R. & Goldberg, G. (1974). *Social service delivery: A structural approach to social work practice.* New York: Columbia University Press.

Miller, P. (1985). Professional use of lay resources, *Social Work.* Sept.-Oct., 409-414.

NiCarthy, G., Merriam, K. & Coffman, S. (1984). *Talking it out: A guide to groups for abused women.* Seattle, WA: The Seal Press.

Pancoast, D., Parker, P. & Froland, C. (1983). *Rediscovering self-help: Its role in social care.* Beverly Hills: Sage Publishers.

Papell, C. & Rothman, B. (1966). Social group work models: Possession and heritage, *Education for Social Work*, 2 (2), 67-77.

Parry, Scott (1979). *Using role playing for group instruction.* New Jersey: Training House, Inc.

Parry, Scott & Robinson, E. (1981). *Participative techniques of group instruction.* New Jersey: Training House, Inc.

Perlman, Helen H. (1979). *Relationship: The heart of helping people.* Chicago: The University of Chicago Press.

Sarason, S.B. (1974). *The psychological sense of community: Prospects for a community psychology.* San Francisco: Jossey-Bass.

Silverman, P.R. (1980). *Mutual aid groups.* Beverly Hills: Sage Publishers.

Trabue, Donna (1988). A model for a mutual help support group for teen mothers. An unpublished manuscript.

Vorrath, H. & Brendtro, L. (1985). *Positive peer culture.* New York: Aldine De Gruyter Publishers.

Wasserman, H. & Danforth, H. (1988). *The human bond: Support groups and mutual aid.* New York: Springer Publishing Company.

The Tasks and Skills
of the Social Worker Across Stages
# of Group Development

Toby Berman-Rossi

While there are many frames of reference through which to view group experience, there is a high degree of agreement, irrespective of viewpoint, that groups do develop over time (Hare, 1976; Lacoursiere, 1980). The concept of group development concerns itself with how a group as a whole changes over time. The idea of the "whole" is the salient point of departure. This "whole," or "it," while influenced by individual members, has a distinguishable identity. The saying "the whole is greater than the sum of its parts" speaks to this reality.

This process of growth has four noteworthy characteristics (Chin, 1969). First, the stages are orderly and predictable. Though groups vary, their development is more similar than dissimilar. Second, stages are interdependent. The developmental tasks of preceding stages must be handled sufficiently so that the group can move on to the tasks of succeeding stages. These tasks need not be mastered exhaustively, but rather just enough so that they no longer are the central preoccupation of the group. Third, how the group grows and its character at a point in time, can both be defined, e.g., "it" is fragmented; "it" is polarized. And fourth, positive value is associated with movement from one stage to the next.

The literature records many efforts to describe this development. Developmental models of three types are specified: linear-progressive, life-cycle, and pendular (Gibbard, Hartman and Mann, 1974). Each type sees itself as including essential developmental elements. Linear-progressive models have two central tenets: (1) linearity is advanced through an "onwards and upwards" process, and

(2) progression occurs when members "resolve" their dependency relationship with the authority and can move on to using each other as a pivotal feature of their association. In this model, dependence (member to authority relationships) always precedes interdependence (member to member relationships). Representatives of this model include Bennis and Shepard (1956) whose seminal work became the basis for later writing (Babed and Amir, 1978; Tuckman, 1965; Tuckman and Jensen, 1977). The life-cycle model, exemplified by Garland, Jones, and Kolodney (1965), is essentially a linear-progressive model with a final stage of termination. These theorists maintain that all closed membership, time limited models (of which Bennis and Shepard spoke) must deal with separation as a final group task. Their stage designations are: (1) pre-affiliation, (2) power and control, (3) intimacy, (4) differentiation, and (5) separation. The pendular, or recurring cycle model denies the linearity of group development. It argues that central group issues are never really resolved sufficiently. The continuous need to resolve these issues pulls the group in a pendular, rather than linear manner. Movement over time develops through this pendular process (Bion, 1961).

It is the fourth component of group development, that of positive value associated with progression, which especially captures the eye of the social worker. A more highly developed group is better able to satisfy members' needs which originally drew them to the group (Berman-Rossi, 1988). Strengthening the group as a whole becomes a practice strategy designed to assist the group in doing "its" work, namely, the satisfying of members' needs.

Attaching our professional practice tasks to the tasks of the group is consistent with a long group work tradition (Schwartz, 1959). This tradition views the group as a mutual aid system in which the worker's role is to strengthen members to be of help to each other as they pursue common tasks (Schwartz, 1961; Shulman, 1985/86). The worker becomes one of many helping relationships. Fortifying the group as a whole further amplifies the mutual aid process and provides directives for professional action.

Practitioners who understand how groups develop can act with a higher degree of consciousness and skill focused upon assisting groups in their maturation. Knowing how to assist a group in its development demands that we strengthen our comprehension of five interdependent group components: (1) character of group system, (2) character of member behavior, (3) member and collective tasks, (4) tasks of the social worker, (5) the skills of the social worker. These five components are an integral part of every stage of group development.

Using the stage designations defined by Garland, Jones, and Kolodney (1965), (pre-affiliation, power and control, intimacy, differentiation, and separation), this paper will discuss each stage according to these elements. A caution should be noted. The following discussion concerns itself primarily with time-limited, close-ended groups. Each practitioner must individualize the material for his/her group and group members. For instance, the work of Schopler and Galinsky (1984) enables us to understand the different ways open-ended groups mature. In addition, while comparative analyses demonstrate similar dominant patterns across groups, the manner in which individual groups grow is influenced by numerous variables including: race, culture, class, ethnicity, gender, age, and focus of the group. For example, while all mature groups must struggle with Stage 2, power and control, we would expect the way the issues arise, the form of its resolution, and the activity of the worker to differ from group to group. A group of frail, institutionalized older persons might need worker encouragement to express negatives towards him/her, while a group of adolescents in a shelter would be more readily expressive.

Familiarity with each of these stages provides the social worker with a tool for assessment. By understanding normative group development, workers are able to define the ways in which their groups differ. Knowledge of these differences can prompt the worker to become curious about whether there are specific issues towards which they should be directing their attention. These issues may reflect obstacles to group development and therefore can help the worker zero in on important work for the group. Additionally, appreciating a group's stage related capabilities can enhance the skill of the worker in developing demands which are appropriate, for each stage, e.g., as when a worker demands too much intimacy in Stage 1 (pre-affiliation) before relationships among members have developed.

The works of Caple (1978); Garland, Jones, and Kolodney (1965); Gitterman and Shulman (1986); Lee and Swenson (1986); Shulman (1984); and Schwartz (1961) have contributed to the subsequent discussion of integrated stage components.

STAGE I: PRE-AFFILIATION

Phase of Work: Preliminary and Beginning

Character of group system. At this initial stage, the group qua group is non-existent and therefore is a source of stress rather than support to members. The work of the group is unknown and the focus ambiguous. The group is without structure and norms. A climate of trust has yet to be developed. Rules of behavior are individually rather than collectively determined. There are individual rather than collective relationships.

Character of member behavior. Members are unable to see a strong connection between their troubles and the troubles of others thereby increasing a sense of uniqueness and isolation. They have little connectedness and mistrust each other as well as the worker. Mistrust of the worker is based upon previous relationships with authorities. Indirect communication with an approach-avoidance pattern in relationships predominates. Strong societal taboos and norms militate against intimacy and sensitive areas of work. Members are uncertain about their ability to handle the demands they imagine will be made upon them. The worker is tested before the members. Members display a visible need for acceptance and support from the worker as well as a desire to be directed. A familiar structure is desired as a means of diminishing anxiety.

Member and collective tasks. In this initial phase there is a need to develop a collective, specific idea of the work of the group based upon the connection between their need and agency service, whereby individual stakes can be located within the collective agreement. Members must establish an initial division of labor between the worker and themselves so potential benefits and obligations may be more clearly understood. The development of an initial structure for work and a culture in which authenticity and honest communication is the norm becomes important.

Tasks of the social worker. The primary task of the social worker, in the initial stage is to clarify purpose and to arrive at a contract with the members as to the terms of their relationship and the focus of work. As components of this primary task the worker is called upon to tune in and develop a preliminary understanding of what the members may be bringing to this experience. She/he is expected to help define the division of labor between the worker and the members in which respective roles are portrayed. She/he is further expected to contribute to the development of a working understanding among the members as to the terms of the contract highlighting the relationship between members' individual stakes and the stake of the group as a whole. Finally, the worker must draw from members their understanding of why they are there and get feedback on the contractual offer, all the time trying to establish a match between agency and member stakes.

Skills of the social worker. (1) To offer a clear uncomplicated statement about the mutual stake between agency and clients in coming together. (2) To generalize client need in an effort to establish connections among group members. (3) To partialize client need, making concerns understood in their specific meaning. (4) To develop receptivity to veiled client communication by responding to non-verbal and oblique expression. (5) To reach for feedback. (6) To encourage specificity in discussion and call attention to cloudiness of expression. (7) To translate covert messages.

STAGE II: POWER AND CONTROL

Phase of Work: Initial Work Phase, Pre-Intimacy

Character of group system. The group changes dramatically during this stage, moving from a kind of formless, ambiguous entity to a unit with primary concerns about power and control. The group is at its most vulnerable and the potential for dissolution looms the greatest. Rules, norms, and status are as yet undefined and there are few guidelines for the difficult work which must occur if the group is to survive. The group becomes polarized over affective and task issues and is principally divided over the authority and competence of the worker. Polarization threatens its very existence. The atmosphere becomes charged with feelings and ideas expressed in strong terms. As the power and control issue is resolving, interdependence is growing. As interdependence rises the group moves towards greater intimacy in the next stage. Some groups spend little time in this stage, "resolving" the "authority theme" quickly; other groups never move beyond.

Character of member behavior. Members are slowly becoming drawn into the group. Ambivalence among members intensifies as the group becomes a possible source of satisfaction. As this potential increases, criticism of the worker also rises as members begin to slowly understand that if they risk involvement they risk potential disappointment. Members become increasingly impatient and critical of each other, differing on the operation of the group. Status differentials among members become important. Members become competitive with regard to the support of the worker, whose protection is needed and feared due to the inherent dependence. A sense of confidence in the worker feels imperative, yet difficult to achieve, at the beginning of this stage. Members feel anxious and angry by the worker's greater latitude of acceptable behavior. Privately they may understand such freedom is necessary for authentic expression. Members may begin to coalesce around criticism of the worker. The process of "resolving" the authority issue is the first major piece of work for which the members need each other. The worker's competence is challenged.

Member and collective tasks. At this stage, the group has two primary tasks: (1) to further develop into a mutual aid system and (2) to "resolve" its relationship with the worker sufficiently to allow it to move on to the work for which it is gathered. As a developing mutual aid system it must further define a structure for work including norms, rules of behavior, and status differentials and must develop a climate of trust. Members must sustain the intensity of this stage, and must begin to view each other as well as the worker as sources of help.

Tasks of the social worker. The two major tasks of the social worker are, as always, directly linked to the tasks of the group. The worker must help the group develop an effective mutual aid system including: a multiplicity of helping relationships, recognition of obstacles and challenges to mutual aid, firmly establishing the common ground between the individual and the group, conveying faith in the group and a vision as to the possibility of change. Developing a structure for work is an integral part of this mutual aid system. The second major simultaneous task is to: engage the challenge to his/her authority, challenge obstacles to engaging the power of the worker, help the group resolve his/her power and develop sufficient trust so that the true work of the group can proceed.

Skills of the social worker. Skills used during this stage highlight the intimate balance between the group's affective and instrumental tasks. Affective skills include: encouraging the expression of difficult and taboo feelings and issues, particularly negatives towards the worker and the collective enterprise; offering direct support of expression; uncoding coded messages; and reaching inside the silence to encourage exploration of difficult material. Instrumental skills include: pointing to obstacles to mutual aid and encouraging their discussion without becoming infatuated by the process; pointing to the common ground between the individual and the group; pointing out when work is occurring and when it is being avoided; helping members move from the general to the specific; partializing larger problems into smaller units; reinforcing the various ways in which members work, especially the ways in which they help each other.

STAGE III: INTIMACY

Phase of Work: Middle Work Phase

Character of group system. At this point the group qua group is seen as satisfying and there is a significant increase in intimacy in member-to-member relationships. With the worker's authority placed in a viable perspective, members can now devote full attention to satisfying their individual needs and being of help to each other. Consensus becomes important and cohesion increases. An agreed upon structure for work and expression of personal needs begin to appear in an atmosphere in which the worker is viewed more positively. There is a sharp increase in goal orientation. With the more realistic perspective on the worker, members begin to understand that they must work for what they get. For the first time, the group is valued for itself and is to be protected and developed. A climate of trust emerges.

Character of member behavior. During this point there is a sharp increase in personal involvement in the form of greater risking and self-revelation. Members begin listening to each other, become more supportive, give to each other with less ambivalence and view each other and the worker as trustworthy. A new exploration of the function of the group strengthens further investment in the group itself. Members are protective of the group, guard against intrusion, stress positives, and become interested in group events.

Member and collective tasks. The group's primary task is to use the growing positive perception of the worker and of each other, to move directly towards the work of the group. Having previously resolved whether it would continue, it now must develop into a need satisfying entity and actually begin to satisfy individual need. Its charge is now to build upon the resolution of the previous stage, of power and control, to develop increasing comfort with and acceptance of more intimate relationships. The possibility of intimacy within the group demands that members invest strongly both in their own situations and those of others. Members are likely to make increased demands of each other.

Tasks of the social worker. As the group begins to operate in its more intimate atmosphere the worker needs to help with two central tasks: aiding the members in establishing a comfortable balance between self-revelation and their need to maintain some sense of privacy and secondly, assisting with the work itself. Members need additional support for their growing intimacy and need the worker to challenge obstacles to the development of mutual aid, e.g., embarrassment over sharing sensitive material. Increasing the demand for work through a call for specificity in discussion will help the group more meaningfully explore the details of the problems before them.

Skills of the social worker. The worker's skills here are designed to help the group maximize its push towards work. All skills are utilized within a context of pointing the members towards each other and towards strengthening individuals to use the group. The worker is called upon to partialize large problems into smaller units, to make note of multiple themes without abandoning attention to specific themes, to point out connections between parts of experiences, to point to connections between the general and the specific, to call for elaboration of issues while encouraging members direct communication with each other and to encourage members to attach affect to intellect. As obstacles and resistance to the work appear, the worker must call attention to and encourage exploration of what was making the work hard.

STAGE IV: DIFFERENTIATION

Phase of Work: End Work Phase

Character of group system. The group as a working unit is now at its most mature, productive, cohesive stage. It has reached its highest degree of achievement and is strong enough to tolerate difference. Group norms are well established and highly functional. The group maintains a high degree of flexibility though roles, status and structure for work are clearly defined and utilized. A satisfying balance between affective and instrumental foci propels group development. At this point, the group is best able to move beyond its own boundaries and interact with its environment.

Character of member behavior. Mutual aid and its inherent interdependence among members are also at their highest level of development at this point. Relationships among members are strongest, as is the relationship between the worker and the members. All are viewed as individuals and differences among them are maximally accepted. As differentiation occurs there is an increase in functional roles. Differences tend to be resolved by consensus, rather than the exercise of status, authority, and power. A strong viable balance between the needs of the individuals and the needs of the group exists. Members have the sense of having gone through a lot together and have come out strong.

Member and collective tasks. The major task of the group is to build upon the development of intimacy of the previous phase and to allow differentiation and the uniqueness of members to be incorporated into group life. In so doing it will be able to provide for individual need satisfaction for members. Individual members must use this period fully to accomplish work. A sense of the end is faintly in sight.

Tasks of the social worker. Understanding that this is the end of the work phase, the practitioner's central task is to help members clarify needs and gains, define remaining issues for attention and with members, labor towards satisfying those needs before the end of the group. Reinforcing strengths, ways of working, and group process assists the members in their efforts to promote differentiation.

Skills of the social worker. Skills at this point are essentially similar to those used in the stage of intimacy, with the addition of the worker pointing to the connections between the specific and the general. This particular skill is highlighted just prior to separation so members can more readily apply gains to future situations.

STAGE V: SEPARATION

Phase of Work: Transitions and Endings

Character of group system. The group as a whole is affected dramatically by its impending demise. All affective and instrumental processes must now be devoted to disbanding the entity which took such great effort to develop. An eventual state of "grouplessness" must be achieved. The length and power of this stage will be influenced by the kind of group and what the group has meant to members. If positive feelings have been strong, those feelings can counter the sense of loss. If positive feelings have been weak, an experience of loss (of real or desired outcomes) will remain. What has been accomplished and how the group can move to disband become central issues during this period. Members avoid new work and try to retain gains. In the face of loss, an approach-avoidance pattern returns.

Character of member behavior. In the face of the strongest ties in the life of the group, members begin to move apart. An approach-avoidance pattern reappears based upon the strength of relationships and the experience of loss. Feelings of loss may generate anxiety and regression over the breaking of bonds. There is an increase in coded behavior, with movement back and forth among a range of responses. Mutual aid continues ambivalently.

Member and collective tasks. In this final stage, the group must evaluate its work, define any remaining tasks, and realistically attend to whatever is still possible. The group must find a way to dissolve its ties, without dissolving what the group has meant and provided. If appropriate, the group must think through and make connections to new resources for satisfaction. Members must achieve some measure of resolve about what they have achieved and must balance attending to their individual needs and the desire of others to be given too in this ending process. Parting well is particularly important.

Tasks of the social worker. The primary task of the social worker is to help the group evaluate work accomplished, define remaining tasks, and complete as much of the outstanding work as possible. The professional must help the group "let go" and move forward towards new pursuits without abandoning established gains. Helping members understand and use the stages of ending (denial, anger, mourning, and acceptance) assists participants with their final set of tasks.

Skills of the social worker. Skills focusing upon both affective and instrumental aspects of the groups' experience are strongly needed. The worker begins by being aware of the use of time to safeguard space for the ending process. She/he will need to reach for the range of feelings generated by ending; establish connections between the ending process and the work of the group; watch and reach for cues with regard to ending turning covert, coded communication into overt, clear expressions; credit the process and outcome of the group reinforcing future supports; summarize discussion; point to the connections between the specific and the general and identify specific next steps. Through all of this, the worker is called upon to offer her/himself closely, and authentically by sharing feelings, experiences, and thoughts within his/her helping function.

CONCLUSION

The notion that groups develop over time is an idea familiar to most practitioners. Whether known theoretically through the literature or primarily through experience, most workers would agree that groups change as time passes. Stages of group development is thought of as a core concept for practitioners because a more highly developed group is a group better able to satisfy members' needs. As a result, social workers should set their sights on assisting the group as a whole in its development so it in turn can provide strength to the work of the group. Understanding of the following five interdependent components provides a sound knowledge base for these efforts: (1) character of group system, (2) character of member behavior, (3) member and collective tasks, (4) the tasks of the social worker, (5) the skills of the social worker. Each of these stage-related components has been described, providing practitioners with both tools for assessments and directives for action. Social work practice can become strikingly more powerful when informed by this knowledge base.

REFERENCES

Babed, E. and L. Amir. "Bennis and Shepard's Theory of Group Development: An Empirical Examination." *Small Group Behavior.* 9:4 (1978): 477-492.

Bennis, W. and H. Shepard. "A Theory of Group Development." *Human Relations.* 9 (1956): 415-57.

Berman-Rossi, T. (1988) "Empowering Groups Through Understanding Stages of Group Development." Proceedings Ninth Annual Symposium, Association for the Advancement of Social Work with Groups. *Social Work with Groups.* Special Issue.

Bion, W. R. *Experiences in Groups.* New York: Ballantine Books, 1961.

Caple, R. "The sequential Stages of Group Development." *Small Group Behavior.* 9:4 (1978): 470-476.

Chin, R. "The Utility of Systems Models and Developmental Models for Practitioners." In W. Bennis, K. Benne, and R. Chin (eds.) *The Planning of Change.* (2nd ed.), New York: Holt, Rinehart and Winston, 1969.

Garland, J., H. Jones, and R. Kolodney. "A Model for Stages of Development in Social Work Groups." In S. Bernstein (ed.) *Explorations in Group Work: Essays in Theory and Practice.* Boston: Boston University School of Social Work, 1965.

Gibbard, G., J. Hartman and R. Mann. "Group Process and Development." In G. Gibbard, J. Hartman, and R. Mann (eds.) *Analysis in Groups*. San Francisco: Jossey-Bass, 1974.

Gitterman A. and L. Shulman (1986) *Mutual Aid Groups and the Life Cycle*. Itasca, Il.: F. E. Peacock Publishers, Inc.

Hare, A. P. *Handbook of Small Group Research*. (2nd ed.) New York: The Free Press, 1976.

Lacoursiere, R. (1980) *The Life Cycle of Groups*. New York: Human Sciences Press.

Lee, J. and C. Swenson. "The Concept of Mutual Aid." In A. Gitterman and L. Shulman (eds.) *Mutual Aid Groups and the Life Cycle*. Itasca, Il.: F. E. Peacock Publishers, Inc., 1986.

Schopler, J. and M. Galinsky. "Meeting Practice Needs: Conceptualizing the Open-Ended Group." *Social Work with Groups*. 7:2 (1984): 3-19.

Schwartz, W. "Group Work and the Social Scene." In A. J. Kahn (Ed.), *Issues in American Social Work*. New York: Columbia University Press, 1959.

Schwartz, W. "The Social Worker in the Group." In *The Social Welfare Forum*, 1961, Proceedings on the National Conference on Social Welfare. New York: Columbia University Press, 1961.

Shulman, L. (1984) *The Skills of Helping Individuals and Groups*. Itasca, Il.: F. E. Peacock Publishers, Inc.

Shulman, L. "The Dynamics of Mutual Aid." In A. Gitterman, and L. Shulman. (eds.) "The Legacy of William Schwartz: Group Practice as Shared Interaction." *Social Work with Groups*. 8:4 (1985/86): 51-60.

Tuckman, B. "Developmental Sequence in Small Groups." *Psychological Bulletin*. 63 (1965): 384-399.

Tuckman, B. and M. Jensen. "Stages of Small-Group Development Revisited." *Group and Organizational Studies*. 2:4 (1977): 419-427.

Group Work and the Environment:
A Systems Approach

Leonard N. Brown

The history of group work as a developing part of social work affirms its commitment to social issues. The social goals model, a categorization of social group work during its early years (Papell and Rothman 1966), emphasized social values and citizen responsibility to improve the environment. The environment is defined as the various psychological, social, and cultural forces that surround the individual. Coyle's writings, in particular, highlighted social action as a valued professional function (Coyle 1947: 131-180; Coyle 1948). Social action or change is one of the features of social work with groups that distinguishes it from group work practiced by other disciplines. The group as part of residential treatment, where the living situation of the institution is considered the immediate environment, has had a long tradition in social work (Maier 1965) and the more recent work with social networks (Maguire 1983; Moore 1978) continues attention to the environment as a vital connection with the helping process.

From a review of group work literature in different helping professions (Zimpfer 1984), there are some recent writings on the use of networks with groups and a continuation of the longstanding tradition of using milieu therapy or the concept of the therapeutic community within the institutional settings as a major form of patient or resident care. However, except for the social work with groups literature, there is little writing on group work to affect environmental conditions. The social work trend in recent years has been more toward clinical practice with individuals, families, and groups. Social work in settlements and neighborhood centers, where community action is still practiced, remains as one of the few types of agencies to continue the commitment to social change.

A typology of social group work and the environment is being described in this paper as encompassing the different forms of organizational or community engagement. Some writers, such as Garvin, Glasser, Carter, English and Wolfson (1985), Frankel and Sundel (1978), Cnaan and Adar (1987) and Schwartz (1976) describe a methodology for environmental change. Some of their work has been considered in the model being presented. In addition, some systems concepts are being incorporated to provide the conceptual rationale for work with the environment.

PRACTICE MODEL AND SYSTEMS CONCEPTS

The group acts upon and responds to different environments. One such environment is the group itself, which is molded by the values, thinking and behavior of each of its members. These thoughts, feelings and actions have their source in the reference groups of the group members–the formal and informal groupings in society which people can identify with and that influence their behavior. For instance, a religion, family, peer group or social class may provide reference groups for people. The physical and social environment of the group members, including some of these reference groups, will also affect the way participants act and think.

Moore (1983) describes the group-in-situation as the unit of attention in social work with groups. An ecological perspective is suggested as combining the group and its situation, which "recognizes the totality of patterned relationships between organisms and their environment" (p. 23). Extragroup means of influence, proposed by Vinter and Galinsky (1985), is a framework for understanding these environmental factors. They include social roles of members prior to being in the group, the significant persons in their lives, the social systems to which they belong, and the social environment of the group.

The relationship of the group to the environment is a systemic one. The group is a sub-system of one or more environments. For instance, it can be considered a sub-system of the larger agency system. A social action group is also a sub-system of a neighborhood as well as the agency system. Individuals are parts of various systems, including family, peer group, organization and community. Since these systems are influential in affecting one's actions, if the system is modified, it will also have an impact on the person's behavior. However, since there are many systems shaping the person's attitudes and actions, there may be a range of expectations for behavior. For instance, the family and peer group of the adolescent may be espousing different values and forms of behavior. The school may attempt to exercise influence in still another way. The adolescent is pulled in different directions and may be confused by these conflicting pressures to conform. The group can help the person identify and sort out these incongruent messages and make thoughtful choices. The group can also work with the group members to achieve more consistency in the expectations of these various systems, thus lessening the incongruence which may be a contribution to behavior problems. Where systems are more consistent in their expectations and uphold the same kinds of values, it is more likely that changes will be supported and reinforced. In the practice model being proposed, there are phases involving some of these key systems people. For each phase there is a systems explanation for conceptual clarity. The phases and their systems counterparts are as follows:

Phase	*Systems Concept*
Identification of need or problem	Initial boundary
Assessment and planning	Boundary clarification
Selection of planning and action group	Organization and energy
Further involvement	Energy and linkage
Change and stabilization	Leverage and dynamic equilibrium

Identification of Need or Problem

This is what is usually considered the presenting problem, when a person or group identifies a need or problem and seeks help from an agency. It may also be a social problem that is cause for concern by the agency. For organizations, it may be an administrative issue that needs attention.

Even though a group has been meeting for reasons of personal change, there may come a time when environmental problems become just as important. When this occurs, the contract with the group may be redefined to include the larger environmental issues.

System Concept: Initial Boundary

Boundary is defined as the border or limited region where there is more energy interchanges within this defined area than outside of it (Anderson and Carter 1984:24). For purposes of this phase it is a perception of how a problem is being manifested and who is involved in it. It is called the initial boundary because it is the way people first recognize and describe it. The focus of energy is a system of thought as well as an actual occurrence.

Assessment and Planning

Once the need or problem has been presented or recognized as requiring attention, there is further exploration about its meaning and who is part of the problem. This could be a time for mapping of personal networks, as suggested by Maguire (1980), in order to identify potential sources of support. At this time, persons are identified who may be in a position to influence the environment in a positive direction.

The intake interview might be used to focus on what is the presenting problem and examine the fuller implications for the person and those in the immediate surroundings. Some agencies will use a needs assessment, whereby persons are asked about their interests and preferences for certain groups or to rank community problems in order to decide on the use of limited resources. The assessment includes a planning dimension, hopefully in collaboration with the person or group that has brought the need or problem to the attention of the agency.

System Concept: Boundary Clarification

As more information becomes known and feelings are expressed, the original conception of the need or problem may be altered or reframed to look differently. The boundary could be modified to include a different arrangement of people and a changed focus in dealing with the problem. For instance, what at first may have seemed like disruptive behavior in the classroom for a young child has taken on new meaning as information has been gathered. It now appears that the parents, teacher, and playground supervisor are involved in the problem because of their conflicting expectations of the child. Any plan for intervention should include their collaboration so that there are consistent expectations and similar goals to help the child.

Selection of Planning and Action Group

When the environmental issue has been brought up in a treatment or socioeducational group, the planning and action take place within the group itself. The group uses a problem-solving approach to consider the next steps in either changing group member behavior to interact with the environment in a more effective way or to use techniques to modify that part of the environment that seems to be contributing to the problem.

When the identification of the environmental problem is emanating from a person, perhaps as a presenting problem, a group could be formed with others who share an interest or concern about the same kind of problem. One of the purposes of their group would be to resolve this particular issue that brought them together.

The need to deal with community concerns may come from agency staff, interested citizens, government or a business organization. In this type of situation, a planning and action group is formed by the practitioner to clarify the meaning of the problem and work toward change. Persons should be selected for this group who have a strong interest in the problem, represent some diversity in their views, are influential in being able to reach others and accessible in terms of time and commitment.

System Concept: Organization and Energy

Organization means that there is clarity about how a system will work and that its parts are so arranged that there will be the best use of available resources. Energy is motivation, action, charisma, power, and whatever other characteristics might describe forces for change. Anderson and Carter (1984:11) state that "energy derives from a complex of sources including the physical capacities of its members; social resources such as loyalties, shared sentiments, and common values; and resources from its environment." The planning and action group should have the necessary organization and energy to mobilize further effort to accomplish its purposes.

Further Involvement

Since there are often many people affected by an environmental problem, a successful change effort will engage a wider spectrum of key persons who can also participate in problem-solving. These are the persons who may be less accessible at first but no less important. They may be in a position to implement a change of direction or offer resistance. For instance, in response to problems of burnout of nurses in a hospital, the administration supported the formation of stress management groups. Besides helping nurses with personal techniques to lessen stress, the work environment also contributed to strain and needed to be modified. The planning and action group (key administrators) went well in terms of recommending the implementation of the program. However, head nurses on the floors, who were not directly involved in the planning, demonstrated resistance to the stress management groups because of interference with ward routine. These middle management nurses were crucial to the successful implementation of the plan and needed to be involved. This is an example of this next layer of participation that is necessary.

Forming coalitions, whereby groups who have a common interest join together, is another way of increasing involvement and using additional resources. Gentry (1987:49) highlights the need for collaboration, horizontal power distribution, and effective communication as essential elements of stable coalition relationships. In some cases there is also the use of media to stimulate interest and favorable attitudes toward the issue under consideration. During this phase, potential recipients of a service would be involved in further planning. For instance, when planning for a teen-age recreation program in response to adolescent delinquency or under-achievement, some teenagers who would be representative of the intended population should participate so that they can contribute their thinking and action to the development of the intended activities.

Systems Concept: Energy and Linkage

The energy generated by the planning and action group stimulates further interest and involvement. There is continued and expanded energy as more persons commit themselves and take responsibility for implementation of any action proposals. When there is this exchange of energy a process of linkage takes place. Linkage means that there are connections among people in regard to the common pursuit of meeting a need or solving a problem. There is strength and power in this collective activity, especially when these forces for change are moving in the same direction. The linking is what Maguire (1980) describes as making contacts with persons from a client's personal network. He differentiates between association of first order and second order networks, all for the purpose of expanding a helping system for the client.

Change and Stabilization

The support for change takes place through active participation by persons who are affected by the problem. It is expected that with increased communication and clarification about common goals and strategies for implementation, there is support for change. It may occur on at least three levels: personal attitudes and skills to react to the environment in a more effective way; group empowerment and capacities for problem-solving; and environmental restructuring to sustain growth and development of group members or those most affected by a social problem. The patterns of communication and arrangements of relationships in the person/group/environment transaction will be modified in the process, starting with identifying the need or problem, moving to assessment, and then incremental steps of involvement by persons in a position to find solutions.

System Concept: Leverage and Dynamic Equilibrium

Linkage with key persons should activate forces for change. The particular combination of influential persons will provide additional weighting, or leverage, toward meeting needs or solving problems. Lippitt, Watson and Westley (1958) see the person or group as a leverage point to begin this process of change. They use linkage to mean the "connection between the leverage point and other parts or functions of the system" (p. 103).

When change occurs it will mean a new balance of relationships, perhaps in how roles are perceived and performed. This "state of balance or adjustment, typically achieved through opposing actions" is called equilibrium (Chess and Norlin 1988: 126). When the equilibrium is in a new position, rather than returning to a former level, it is called dynamic equilibrium (Chin 1961:205). If there is continued support and reinforcement of these new relationships and structures, it will be maintained. A sufficient number of persons, especially those who have the power to influence decision-making, need to be involved in the change process in order for it to succeed.

GROUPS ORGANIZED IN RELATION TO ENVIRONMENTAL NEED OR PROBLEM

This type of group has social action or system change as its function, although the process of reaching that goal can also have therapeutic effects on the group members and the group as a whole. Being able to effect change in the environment can be an empowering experience, raising self-esteem and contributing to a sense of mastery or control over one's life situation.

The need or problem may be identified by persons, groups, or organizations within the community. The focus for change could be the amelioration or prevention of a social problem, the provision of a new service or the restructuring of an organization. This kind of social work practice has traditionally been the province of community organization. However, the direct practitioner is taking on some aspects of this role as a valid function for prevention and community practice within agencies. It fits in with the model of the generalist social worker.

EXAMPLE

Guidance counselors at a high school became increasingly aware of the difficult adjustment for incoming freshmen to the high school. Many of them had academic problems, felt intimidated by the older students and demonstrated negative behavior in classes. The social worker at the high school talked to the guidance counselors at the high school and middle school to find out more about the problems. He also spoke to some of the freshmen to hear what they had to say. The social worker learned that although there was a large meeting at the middle school to inform the students about high school, the ninth graders had little idea what was expected of them. They became the scapegoats of the older students. In many cases, they felt too young and awkward to participate in extra-curricular activities.

IDENTIFICATION OF PROBLEM: poor school performance and behavior problems
ASSESSMENT AND PLANNING: unclear expectations, low self-esteem, feeling scapegoated

The social worker met with representatives (principals and guidance counselors) from the middle school and high school to discuss the problem and seek solutions. These persons were in a position to make administrative decisions or at least to initiate the possibility of change by involving others at both schools. The idea of a peer leadership program was introduced as one means of dealing with the problem. This would involve junior and senior students as support persons to the freshmen. It was envisioned as something like a big brother and big sister program.

PLANNING AND ACTION GROUP: key persons from middle school and high school; considering systemic as well as student aspects of problem

To become more fully engaged in planning and implementation, this initial administrative group brought together other persons to sound them out on the proposed plan. This larger group included students from the high school and middle school, other guidance counselors and some teachers who were particularly interested in the concept of peer support.

FURTHER INVOLVEMENT: wider array of participants, more diversity in group composition

Interested sophomore and junior students were recruited and participated in a series of training sessions, including a week-end away from school at a camp. Each peer leader was assigned to a small group of freshmen. The role of the peer leader was defined as providing a helping relationship with ninth grade students in the areas of academic enrichment, recreation and socialization, and referral to school or community activities. Training sessions continued for the peer leaders to deal with issues and problems in their relationships with the younger students.

In an evaluation of the program using a standardized instrument (Jesness Behavior Checklist), there were positive findings in all the measurable characteristics of behavior compared to a control group. There were also parent groups, family treatment and a professionally led counseling group for some of the freshmen. It was found that the peer leaders also benefitted greatly from the overall experience.

CHANGE AND STABILIZATION: enhanced self-image, more active in school activities, improved academic work

In this illustration, the social worker starts with the broader social and behavioral problem–poor school performance and behavior problems by ninth grade students. Although it is certainly necessary to individualize for each of these pupils in regard to their specific needs and problems, the environment of the middle school and high school are considered as part of the broader problem. The schools have the potential to be part of the solution as well. In this way the boundary of the problem is re-conceptualized to include the school environment. Once the planning and action group meets they clarify the problem according to the broader context of the student/environment transaction. Within this framework an array of solutions is sought. Persons are involved as part of a helping network. The idea of a peer leadership program is one of the consequences of this kind of thinking. Other possibilities include preparation of parents to offer specific kinds of supportive help, in-service training of ninth grade teachers, after school academic enrichment classes or a series of meetings while the pupils are still in the eighth grade regarding expectations for the high school. There might also be support/socialization groups led by guidance counselors. Combinations of the above possibilities would be useful. In all these approaches the child is not singled out as the problem. Conceptualizing the problem within an interactional pattern of the child and his or her social situation is consistent with the notion of social work with groups. When the pupil is not burdened with a deviant label, the environment will contribute to a healthier self-image and enable the child to join in helping efforts as a collaborator rather than a victim.

It was mentioned in the illustration that the peer leaders (juniors and seniors) benefited greatly from this experience. It enabled them to take on the role of helper and was a step in the transition to adulthood. The training and participation with the ninth graders emphasized the use of their strengths and raised their self-esteem. They learned problem-solving skills which will be beneficial in their everyday life. The advantage for the peer leaders as helping persons is also true for others who are mobilized to provide support, energy, and resources to those in need. The fact that the helpers are helped tends to be overlooked. While the purpose of their involvement is not to enrich them personally, this often happens. They become more socially conscious citizens and resourceful helpers for others.

The group worker takes on more of the coordinator role, emphasizing adequate communication and facilitating linkages. The worker recognizes the importance of organization–the system term for clarity of purposes, roles, and the accompanying structure–and energy to generate interest and ideas. The concept of linkage, perhaps using coalitions or helping people join together, is basic to resolving social problems in the environment. The persons in the planning and action group are influential enough to exercise leverage in the linking process. An important reason to involve key administrative or community persons who are part of the target for change is that their power will assure more stability of change, since they have been involved in decision-making about solutions.

CONCLUSIONS

Group work in the environment moves toward further integration of social work in direct practice and community organization. It can apply to work with families, small groups, residential living, organizations or communities. The methodology that was outlined in this chapter seems to be applicable in all of these situations. One of the differences in this model that is not always considered in direct practice is the notion of "further involvement." This is meant to be the involvement of persons who are potentially supportive in the lives of clients or in being able to influence change in the environment. They represent a vast reservoir of resources, often untapped or underutilized. Indigenous leadership is most often associated with this phase.

The roles for the social worker who is engaged in environmental change are more varied than in any other type of practice. He or she might be mediator, educator, advocate, broker, therapist, consultant, or coordinator. It requires a good knowledge of resources that are related to the need or problem and when to use them. The social worker might use the power, control, and authority of his or her position but must be prepared to share it with the broadening base of persons who are willing to take responsibility for planning and implementing action proposals. It is only as others can exercise influence that change will occur. Empowerment is very much at the heart of group work in the environment.

REFERENCES

Anderson, R.E. and Carter, I. (1984). *Human Behavior and the Social Environment* (3rd ed.). New York: Aldine.
Chess, W.A. and Norlin, J.M. (1988). *Human Behavior and the Social Environment: A Social Systems Model.* Boston: Allyn and Bacon.

Chin, R. (1961). The Utility of System Models and Developmental Models for Practitioners. In W.G. Bennis, K.D. Benne & R. Chin (Eds.), *The Planning of Change* (pp. 201-214). New York: Holt, Rinehart and Winston.

Cnaan, R.A. and Adar, H. (1987). An Integrative Model for Group Work in Community Organization Practice. *Social Work with Groups*, 10 (3), 5-24.

Coyle, G.L. (1947). *Group Experience and Democrative Values*. New York: Woman's Press.

Ephross, P.H. and Vassil, T.V. (1988). *Groups that Work*. New York: Columbia University Press.

Frankel, A.J. and Sundel, M. (1987). The Grope for Group: Initiating Individual and Community Change. *Social Work with Groups*, 1 (4), 399-405.

Garvin, C.D., Glasser, P.H., Carter, B., English, R. and Wolfson, C. (1985). Group Work Intervention in the Social Environment. In M. Sundel, P. Glasser, R. Sarri and R. Vinter (Eds.), *Individual Change Through Small Groups* (pp. 277-293). New York: Free Press.

Gentry, M.E. (1987). Coalition Formation and Process. *Social Work with Groups*, 10 (3), 39-54.

Lippitt, R., Watson, J. and Westley, B. (1958). *The Dynamics of Planned Change*. New York: Harcourt, Brace and World.

Maguire, L. (1980). The Interface of Social Workers With Personal Networks. *Social Work with Groups*, 3 (3), 39-49.

_____, (1983). *Understanding Social Networks*. Beverly Hills, CA: Sage.

Maier, H.W. (Ed.). (1965). *Group Work as Part of Residential Treatments*. New York: National Association of Social Workers.

Moore, E.E. (1978). The Implications of System Network for Social Work With Groups. *Social Work with Groups*, 1 (2), 133-143.

_____, (1983). The Group-in-Situation as the Unit of Attention in Social Work With Groups. *Social Work with Groups*, 6 (2), 19-31.

Schwartz, W. (1976). Between Client and System: The Mediating Function. In R.W. Roberts and H. Northern (Eds.), *Theories of Social Work With Groups* (pp. 171-197). New York: Columbia University Press.

Vinter, R.D. and Galinsky, M.H. (1985). Extragroup Relations and Approaches. In M. Sundel, P. Glasser, R. Sarri, and R. Vinter (Eds.), *Individual Change Through Small Groups* (pp. 266-276). New York: Free Press.

Zimpfer, D.G. (1984). *Group Work in the Helping Professions* (2nd ed.). Muncie, IN: Accelerated Development.

A Social Group Work Model
for Latency-Aged Children
from Violent Homes

Doug Evans
Wendy Shaw

There is increasing research that recognizes that children who live in homes where there is violence between their parents are children vulnerable to physical, social and psychological problems.[1] Studies indicate that a high percentage of abusive husbands have been child-witnesses to parental domestic violence.[2] Our experience with assaulted women's groups indicate that many adult victims of domestic violence were also child-witnesses to parental domestic violence. It seems clear that services to children can play a primary role in breaking the cycle of family violence, as well as serve to help the children with their current functioning.

Recent research has established common symptomatologies among children from violent homes.[3] Because of the common problems experienced by these children group intervention programs are a logical therapeutic approach. The paradigm of most of the research is social learning theory. The group programs established in Ontario[4] are also based on social learning theory. These programs have established group outlines that are designed to help the children label feelings, develop safety plans, understand domestic violence, and learn problem-solving skills. The themes and exercises suggested in these group program manuals are excellent. However, the programs are limited by their short-term, educational approach. They do not utilize the strengths brought to the group by each child. Nor do they utilize the group setting's potential for "mutual support and mutual challenge."[5] Such utilization can only be accomplished by considering group process and incorporating it into the group program.

During the past four years we have been developing therapeutic domestic violence programs for latency-aged children at a family counselling agency in Toronto.* Our model is based on: (1) our knowledge of groups and group process; (2) our understanding of the clinical issues and dynamics related to family violence; (3) activities from the New Beginnings Manual[6] and (4) media from social skills development group literature.

In the following paper we will explore the limitation of educational models. We will describe a social group work model of intervention for children from violent homes, and will illustrate how such a model better addresses their needs.

CURRENT GROUP WORK MODELS DESIGNED TO TREAT CHILDREN EXPOSED TO DOMESTIC VIOLENCE

Treatment models in use in Ontario tend to be educational in orientation. Their purpose is to teach the children more functional ways of understanding and dealing with the confusing, painful, and dangerous family situations to which they may be subjected. The groups are only ten sessions or less in length. Each session is based upon a pre-determined theme such as separation, understanding family violence, or feelings. They rarely devote more than a portion of a single session to any of these topics. Because the agenda for the group as a whole and for individual session is predetermined by the model it does not reflect the individual needs of group members or the issues that arise in the formation of a group. The new ways of interacting taught by these programs reflect a series of values which, however much more functional they may be, are often completely contradictory to those of the child's most important relational sys-

---

* We have also utilized the model for a group of children aged five to seven. Although the curriculum was modified to reflect their cognitive abilities and developmental stage and the group process opportunities were somewhat limited, the model worked very successfully. The model is currently being applied to groups for adolescents from violent homes, again with modifications to reflect cognitive and developmental stages. For the purposes of the paper, however, "children" will denote latency-aged children only.

tem–his or her family. The models leave no time for dealing with the confusion or the loyalty issues that such a contradiction naturally raises. In the educational models very little time, if any, is devoted to dealing with the interrelations between group members, between the group leaders and the children and between the leaders themselves. This is a major weakness of the models because the difficulties these children present with are often a result of relationship problems.

Educational models, by attempting to teach children new, more functional relationship and interpersonal skills, while ignoring the relationship and interpersonal issues which inevitably arise in groups, end up presenting their group members with a paradox, "Do as we say, not as we do!"

Our Experiences Using Educational Models

Our pilot groups for children from homes where there is domestic violence were based upon the short-term educational models developed in Ontario. We experienced difficulties that seemed directly attributable to the models' inherent paradox resulting from not utilizing group process. The commitment of the group members to the group was problematic. The children's responses to the exercises and interventions often seemed superficial. They often appeared to express what they felt would please the group leaders rather than their real feelings.

Our intake procedure was inadequate and we felt that we had to rethink the issues of group composition and duration. Endings, so very important to these children who frequently have histories of troubled endings, needed to be dealt with more sensitively and effectively. We felt that we needed to be far more aware of the needs and issues of both individual members and of the group as a whole. We felt that we had to understand the issues between us, as co-leaders, so that we could effectively use our relationship and skills to help the group process. This feeling was based on our strong conviction that the manner in which co-leaders handle the issues that arise in their team gives a subtle, but powerful, message that could reinforce dysfunctional stereotypes and interactional patterns.

We believed that we had to continually address our own responses to domestic violence and how these responses were influencing the group. If we did not look at our values objectively we risked expressing them unconsciously and indirectly. Negative patterns of indirect communication are common problems for many of these children and leader behaviour could serve to reinforce those very patterns which we were trying to change.

Our conclusion from our groups based on the educational model was that we needed to consider the group's process as well as the program content. In subsequent groups we have changed our approach to include group process and development. In planning the group we have addressed the issue of group goals, size, duration, composition, and leadership. We have devised an intake and pre-group affiliation process. Through our own study of groups and with the aid of a consultant we have explored the process and developmental stage of our groups in order to effectively plan both individual sessions and the group as a whole. We have explored the issues that have developed between us, as co-leaders in the group. Lastly, we have facilitated a therapeutic ending phase, the phase which is particularly neglected in the educational models.

Although we have not had the opportunity to have our group formally evaluated, responses from the children, schools, parents, and colleagues have confirmed our subjective observations that our new model is better than the educational models at addressing the core problems of these children.

The Pre-Group Planning Phase

The goals of a therapeutic group for children from violent homes are twofold. First, the group needs to help its members develop essential safety skills. They need to know how to respond during times of crisis or potential violence in the family. They need to learn how to stay out of the physical battles between their parents. And, they need to learn that the fighting is not their fault. Second, the group needs to help the children with the behavioural and interactional problems they are experiencing. To address the first goal we continued to rely on the curriculum from the educational models that addressed safety needs. To address the second goal of the therapeutic needs of the children, we utilized social group work technology to develop a mutual aid process.

In order to foster the mutual aid process a group ideally consists of only five to seven members. To facilitate interaction the members should be at a similar level of development. Similar chronological age is helpful, but not essential. To allow the mutual aid process adequate time to take place the group needs to be at least twenty weeks in duration.

Since most of the symptomatic difficulties experienced by the group members are connected to dysfunctional family situations, the group, we believe, should replicate a family system. Our groups, as a result, are co-educational and co-lead by a male and female leadership team. For the purposes of continuity we chose a closed group format. However, there may be circumstances, for example a shelter setting, where open membership would make sense.

Screening and Intake

As with any group it is important that all potential group members are screened. Screening addresses two questions: (1) whether group intervention is a useful treatment for the child and, (2) whether the particular group, as it is constituted, will be able to meet this child's needs. Part of the assessment includes the level of emotional and behavioural disturbance. In order to answer the foregoing questions we convene with the child, his or her custodial parent(s), the family's referring worker, and one group leader. It is essential that both the group leaders and the family understand how the group would fit into an overall plan dealing with the issues that have arisen from the violence in the home and with the child's particular difficulties.

The intake interview is the beginning of the group for each child. For the children we are treating this meeting is frequently the first open discussion of the violence and problems in their homes that they have ever experienced. The manner in which we approach the secret of violence sets a tone that has a significant impact upon the child's future participation in the group. The intake interview must model both sensitivity and directness. Our understanding of the issues, feelings, myths, and fears of children from these homes is our greatest tool. We confront the secret that there is, or has been, violence in their family. We help the child understand and articulate how the violence has affected them personally. We help them identify the problem they have that the group may help them with. The child is helped to see that he or she and other children with similar histories and difficulties can help each other in the group.

We underline that violence will be discussed in the group and establish a bond of confidentiality. We are open about exceptions to confidentiality, such as when we are legally responsible to report abuse. In these families violence has usually been a long and well-kept secret. It is often difficult for the parent(s) to support a confidential group for their child. It evokes fears of disclosure for parents and issues of loyalty for their child. These feelings and fears must be confronted openly.

Finally, the child is helped to articulate, as far as he or she is able, goals for themselves within the group.

It is crucial that the contract for the child's participation in the group include all the parties attending the intake interview. We often meet these children at a very destabilized period in their family's lives. They may be living in temporary shelters. Parents may be going through periods of depression and immobility. All must make commitments to their roles in ensuring the child's regular attendance. It is often necessary to discuss how to deal with potential difficulties. The plan often needs to include the family's support workers.

By the end of a thorough intake the child and his or her family understand the group's purpose, how it fits their needs, and how it connects to other services. The child has made an initial connection with one of the leaders and has talked of what use the group can be for him or her. The child, parent(s), and their worker understand, and have agreed to, their parts in the group. Regular attendance and full participation in the group is far more likely having elicited these understandings and, therefore, the potential for benefitting the child is far greater.

The Initial Sessions

The first day of any new experience is anxiety producing for all of us. The first time members attend a group is fraught with fear and ambivalence. This is a phenomenon well-documented by group work theory and obvious to anyone who has ever lead or participated in a group. For the children who attend our groups, however, the first sessions are laden with negative feelings. The group's purpose, to talk about the violence within their families and the feelings this violence engenders, usually violates a strong family taboo with which the child has lived for his or her entire life. Although at least one parent has supported the group the children have realistic fears about the consequences their disclosures may have in their family or in larger systems like the law, for example.

Many of these children have had little or no experience of truly supportive relationships. They have protected themselves by isolating themselves. The group takes this "solution" away from them. Some children have had miserable experiences with peers. For them the other children participating in the group constitute a real threat. These situations have led us to expect a great deal of fear and ambivalence from group participants. We have found that we must really "tune into" what is going on behind the scenes as these children often do not directly express their feelings. It is insufficient for the children to merely know that they share similar histories and, perhaps, similar problems. They need to understand that their intense feelings about starting in the group are universal, normal, and accepted by everyone.

We have found that the time it takes our groups to go through the tasks of the beginning stage can be quite extended. The members are children who frequently equate relationships with violence, who have found security in silence and isolation, who have known no place, especially not their home, that is safe. They must, therefore, be convinced that the group is a safe place. They must be guaranteed that their disclosures and behaviour will be kept within the confines of the group. They must be coaxed into reaching out and beginning to make connections with other group members and with the leaders. The pace at this stage must, of necessity, be very slow.

Often the children will test the safety of the group or the genuineness of relationships by acting up in the group. They may verbally or physically abuse another member or gang up on or exclude a member in a hurtful way. The leaders must expect this. They need to understand that these behaviours are expressions of natural fear and ambivalence and must help the members come to this understanding themselves. The leaders must act to keep the group safe and must emphasize their interventions as having this ultimate goal. The leaders need to help the members understand how they must all be responsible to each other in that respect.

We have found that our group takes at least three or four sessions before the members are able to successfully accomplish the begin tasks of understanding the group's purpose, setting their own rules for the group, and establishing routines before moving on to the "work" of the group.

As part of the beginning phase it is extremely important for the children to set goals for themselves in the group. In the first session the children should be encouraged to talk about the violence in their own home with one another. We find that they are usually very curious about this aspect of one another's lives. They may be, to a degree, open to admitting that their own parents fight and how that affects them. They may talk about how they have been physically hurt in parental battles. While much of this discussion seems to occur spontaneously we must remind ourselves that such admissions represent a real risk for each child. As leaders we must validate that risk and underscore the importance of confidentiality for the whole group. Talking about their own problems is much harder for the children. Often the children most open to discussing their families find that, at this point, they have nothing to say. Others may talk about superficial or vague difficulties or goals.

As leaders we usually are aware of each child's particular problems. We must remember, however, that the difficulty these children experience setting goals is far greater than just the risk of talking about their problems. It is also an expression of their ambivalence about making a connection with and a commitment to the group. Building the level of trust and security essential to making such a commitment to any group is time consuming. For these children, who have such hurtful associations with relationship and commitment, building trust is an extremely slow process. As leaders our patience and understanding is critical. It models patience and understanding for the group. Such a climate is the foundation of our groups' cohesion. As the process proceeds the children become increasingly able to articulate genuine goals and to make agreements together, helping each other to make important changes in their lives. These goals are the connections that become the life-blood of the group.

The children in our groups care deeply about one another. To a greater degree, however, they care about The Group. They quickly come to compromises and will take great risks for The Group. The children's own goals become invaluable tools to us, as leaders, through the stormy, conflictual stage of the group. The children are motivated by their own goals to find new non-violent means of solving problems.

They are also committed to helping one another to do so. Mutual aid possibilities are abundant.

The Conflict Stage

The middle phase of group development is characterized by conflict. It is "the struggle between the group's primitive instincts to avoid the pain of growth and its need to become more sophisticated and deal with feelings."[7] Bion describes this process as "fight vs. flight."[8] The issues in this stage of group development often parallel the issues in the violent marital relationships of the children's families. In these marriages fighting to resolve conflict and withdrawing to avoid conflict are common themes. Abusers have not developed the capacity to express painful emotions such as jealousy or sadness. Instead, the emotion becomes expressed as anger that intensifies to levels of abuse. The unspoken or spoken family rule is that no one confronts the abuser. The female victims of violence also do not express painful affect directly. Anger towards their partner may be suppressed, scapegoated, or approached indirectly, i.e., through nagging. The children also play a role in these dysfunctional structures. They learn not to express affect directly, but rather to respond to conflict with aggression or by withdrawal. These behaviours become their communication of feelings even though they are not consciously connected to their affect. It is this indirect expression of feelings that creates many of the problems these children present.

Group leaders can unknowingly and unconsciously recreate in their groups the very dynamics that have occurred in the families of the children in the group. One leader may respond to the "mothering" needs of the group. They may help avoid or diffuse conflict in the group–between the children, the children and the other leader, or the co-leaders themselves. The second leader may act more as the disciplinarian and be more task focussed. They may overpower their co-leader in team decisions. These kinds of dynamics can be so subtle that the leaders may not be aware of them. However, the children will be intensely aware of such undercurrents. They may be very familiar to them from their own family's interactions. In fact, the children often recreate the dynamics of their families in the group to enable themselves to function in a familiar environment.

As an example, during one group session, the female leader was absent. The children were thrilled when the male leader brought donuts for a snack, a change from the nutritional snacks the female leader had been providing. The male leader joked about doing this. The following week one of the children secretly informed the female leader of what the male leader had brought to the group, expressing concern about how wrong it had been, and expecting the female leader to be upset. This child easily slid into a triangulating relationship, a natural pattern from her own family. Rather than reinforcing this coalition the female leader mentioned the donuts to the male leader, in front of the group. An interesting discussion ensued that connected the situation to families. This direct communication was different for the child and other group members, who expressed surprise at the process. The following session, when cheese and crackers were served, the children joked about the nutritional snack. At first glance this may seem an insignificant gain but the little girl involved made a fundamental change in how she dealt with conflict. Later experiences in the group gave her the opportunity to practice and expand her ability to deal with conflict openly.

The leaders require each other's support at this stage in order to be effective. If they undermine one another, even in subtle ways, the group is sure to react. The group leaders may become immobilized fearing to "take a side." The children may act out their confusion. This behaviour will likely be interpreted as being related to the domestic violence or to behavioural problems when it is actually mirroring the "battle" between the leadership team.

In order to effectively resist the triangles that the children will attempt to impose on the group the leaders need to find ways to objectively look at how they themselves function as a team. Open discussion between sessions is essential. The use of video tape recordings of the group can serve to enhance the leaders' objectivity. The perspective of a third party, such as a colleague, a group work supervisor, or a consultant, can also be really helpful.

During the conflict stage the children will engage in patterns of behaviour that they have learned from their own families. They may become aggressive, bullying, abusive, and defiant or they may isolate themselves, refuse to participate, and cling to the leaders. Leaders may be tempted to respond by punishing or protecting the child. If leaders respond to behaviours as behaviours in isolation they are responding to, and therefore, reinforcing, indirect communication. The leaders need to identify the behaviours as communication. They can then help the child to express himself more directly to the group and can help the group respond to that communication more appropriately.

During the process of re-directing conflict the tension in the group builds. The children may try to diffuse this tension in various ways, for example, by physically leaving the discussion, suggesting that the group play a game, or by talking about how boring the group is. The leaders also feel this intense level of tension. It is tempting to cooperate with the group members who are attempting to diffuse tensions, or even, at times, to initiate diffusion tactics themselves.

There is no right or wrong answer for how to deal with tension in the group. What is important is that the leaders understand what the function of the tension is in individual and group development and that they help the group to understand this. The following excerpt from one of our groups will illustrate the process of helping the group deal with tension.

First Group Member: This is boring. Let's play a game.

Second Group Member: Yeah, let's play a game.

Leader: Fighting is tough stuff to talk about, but it's what you're here to talk about.

Second Group Member: But it's boring.

Leader: If we stop talking about it, is it because it's boring or because it's so hard to talk about.

Second Group Member: Because it's hard to talk about . . . but I still want to play a game.

First Group Member: I want to play a game.

Leader: Doug [the other leader] and I understand that this is difficult to talk about. We also believe that it will be helpful for you to talk about fighting. If the group decides to play a game now, it doesn't mean that we won't come back to talking about fighting. But sometimes, when feelings are too painful, it is okay to leave them for awhile.

Leader to Co-Leader: I think it should be the group's choice whether we continue the discussion or play a game. What do you think?

Co-Leader: I agree, it's the group's choice.

Third Group Member: Let's play the game, but then we'll come back [to the discussion] before the snack.

After further discussion among the children they agree to the Third Member's suggestion. Not only have they understood the diffusion tactic but they have had the opportunity to actually resolve a problem, for which they received positive reinforcement. The group realized they could make decisions that overrule the leaders. This empowered them and supported the mutual aid process.

In our model group agendas are planned based upon both the needs of the individual children and on the group's phase of development. As the group progresses the leaders become less and less central. The planning focusses less on program content and more on interventions related to the member's interactional patterns and group process. Group themes and homework assignments are utilized. Often the homework introduces an issue or theme for problem-solving but it acts only as a catalyst for the group's discussion. The content of the homework may quickly become unimportant as illustrated by the following example: As a very quiet, unassertive child was presenting his homework to the group the other children began to talk.

Leader to First Group Member: Do you think anyone is listening to you?

First Group Member: No.

Leader: You have a problem. You're talking, but no one is listening. What can you do about that?

First Group Member: I don't know.

Leader: What can you do if you don't know?

First Group Member: Ask the group?

The leader encourages the First Group Member to do so.

First Group Member to Group: Why isn't anyone listening to me?

Second Group Member: Because you talk so quietly we can't hear.

Third Group Member: And you're boring. You go on and on.

Leader: That's good advice. Could you try to show us your work again and make use of those suggestions?

First Group Member: Okay.

The First Group Member then starts again, this time trying to incorporate the suggestions of the group into his presentation.

In the above example learning about problem-solving became experiential rather than cognitive.

As the group matures the members become increasingly able to set their own agendas and to maintain focus on their own. The leaders have to recognize when the group is able to take on these responsibilities and begin to act more as resources to the group. If they continue to remain central at this stage the leaders risk undermining the autonomy the children have gained. Such autonomy is fundamental to the childrens' ability to take their skills outside the group.

Ending the Group

Group endings are difficult and painful for any of us. They evoke previous endings experienced in life and the feelings associated with those endings. A group leader's personal and professional experiences with endings influences how the leader perceives and deals with them. There is a strong tendency for the leaders themselves to deny, shorten, or avoid endings.

This population of children have often experienced many tragic, painful, and confusing endings. Multiple and abrupt separations between their parents result in frequent moves and the many adjustments that have resulted from moving, i.e., school changes and loss of friends. Due to the violence in their homes many of these children have not had the opportunity to say goodbye to their fathers, because their mothers have been forced to secretly move into shelters in the middle of the night or while their spouses are at work. It is difficult for the children to talk about the loss of their father because of the pain it evokes for them.

Educational models deal with endings in a dysfunctional manner. In these models, only the last meeting is devoted to endings. The "ending" is encapsulated in prescribed exercises, designed to encourage expression of feeling about endings. These exercises rely solely on verbal or written expression of feelings, but children often express feelings behaviourally. This population of children find it especially difficult to articulate feelings of hurt or sadness. This task-oriented approach sets up a lack of genuineness. The answers are often superficial or surface responses.

During the intake process, the children contract for a specific number of group sessions that make up the duration of the group. The worker discusses with the parents and the children the importance of completing the group. An important part of the screening process is to help the family assess the reality of their ability to make such a commitment. It is also contracted that if a child must leave the group, it is important for the child and the group, that the child have the opportunity to say goodbye to the group members. This discussion of ending prior to the group even beginning helps the family begin to understand the importance of endings and is an opportunity to discuss other endings in their lives. The group can be seen as an opportunity to "end" differently.

Ending is discussed again at various times during the group's existence. Throughout the course of the group, the children are encouraged to be aware of how many sessions there are in total and the number of sessions remaining. Due to frequent moves and the common pattern of returning home to the abuser, it is realistic to expect that sometimes children will not be able to complete the group. When this happens, parents are encouraged to allow their child to say goodbye to the other group members. The loss of a group member is an opportunity to help the remaining members begin to connect to their own feelings about loss and endings. The leaders can facilitate such connections, and can discuss their own feelings as related to both the loss of the group member and to the eventual ending of the group.

The ending phase which takes place in the last few sessions of the group does have distinctive dynamics which necessitate specific leadership understandings and skills. "The ending phase offers the greatest potential for powerful and important work."[9] In our model we usually begin to address ending at about the fourth to last session. At this point the group members have begun to engage in the regressive behaviours common to this phase. The job of the leaders is to help the group understand this behaviour as the expression of their feelings about ending. The leaders normalize the behaviours and assure the children that previous groups have experienced similar dynamics. They then encourage members to express their feelings verbally and in a more functional manner.

Strong feelings at the point of ending with the children in our groups is to be expected because for many of them it is the most supportive, safe environment that they have ever experienced. The connection of the group's ending to abandonments in their own past is inevitable. For many members there are feelings of disappointment; a feeling that the group is ending before it really had an opportunity to get going. They may feel that they have been unable to accomplish their goals.

Accepting the group's anger and dealing with their often extreme behaviours at this stage is particularly demanding for the leaders. As discussed, they have their own issues and emotional responses to endings. These feelings are often compounded in groups with these children by the leaders' sense of the children's fragility and fears about the hostile environments to which they will be returning. The urge to deny or "smooth over" these very painful issues can be almost irresistible.

It is at this point that co-leaders and supportive supervisors, consultants, or peers can be most important. They can help the group leaders to express and accept their own reactions to the ending process. The leaders can then better separate their own issues from the those of the group and can more objectively deal with the behaviours in the group, redirecting the group members to look at their own pain and fears, and helping them through the process. Only then can the members recount their successes, look realistically at their own strengths, and look ahead to "life after The Group."

In our model the children play a major role in planning their ending. They plan a celebration which takes place at the last group session. The ending phase discussions are completed prior to the last session. The last session is a celebration of knowing each other. It is too late to deal with unfinished business. Leaders must be prepared to assert these boundaries in appropriate ways. For example, in one of the groups, during the second last session, the children began a fight which ended up involving the whole group. Several children were hurt. The leaders had to intervene and physically restrain the children. Immediately afterwards, the leaders helped the children to connect the fighting to their feelings about ending the group. The children began to discuss their sadness intensely. They were crying and huddling close together. This was a powerful, spontaneous event that had an impact on everyone involved. Following this discussion the group was able to plan a bowling party for their final meeting, a task that they had been unable to accomplish during the previous two sessions. They also talked about the school and neighbourhood friends with whom they would be involved at the scheduled group time after the last meeting. The leaders successfully helped the children to connect their feelings to other endings in their lives.

CO-TERMINUS GROUPS FOR CHILDREN AND MOTHERS OF VIOLENT FAMILIES

At the family counselling agency we have run groups for the mothers of the children in our groups. The idea was suggested by Sinclair in her manual *Understanding Wife Assault*.[10] These groups are run in the same building, at the same time as those for the children. Most of the mothers in the group had previously been involved in support groups for abused women or battered wives. This group differed in that it is focussed more upon the women's issues as mothers rather than on issues of violence.

This experiment has had several advantages for both groups. Many children from violent homes are extremely protective of and worried about their very vulnerable, hurting mothers. They have frequently sacrificed their own needs in their efforts to "prop up mom." Furthermore, the way in which they have helped their mothers have frequently been part of dysfunctional family interactions which may reverse family hierarchy or impede the children's moving out into the world of their peers. For the children whose mothers participated in the mother's group knowing that their mothers were being taken care of elsewhere seemed to free them to deal with their own issues and to help themselves. Often, when the children would bake or cook or make crafts as an activity in the group they would take their products as gifts to the mothers in the group. This seemed to us a more functional way to support a parent than the ways often practiced in the family.

The children's group was frequently a struggle for the children. They often left the group saddened or highly charged by the affects evoked during the session. As members of their own group the mothers seemed to have a better understanding of the effects of participating in a therapeutic group. At times when they could not understand their children's worrisome behaviours or affect the children's group leaders were readily available to assist them. Issues did not fester or escalate but were, rather, confronted promptly and appropriately.

It is very disempowering to a parent to have to surrender to someone else the responsibility for dealing with important problems in your child's life. The mothers in the group were able to support the children's group in significant ways, for example, as customers for bake sales, or by participating in the Christmas lunch. Their contributions to the children's group were noticed by the children. This notice had the effect of reinforcing the mothers' sense of competence and their value as a parent. They always seemed invigorated following the times when the two groups interacted.

Often the homework assignments for the group, for example, interview Mom about her past, bringing in a piece of family memorabilia, or drawing a picture of doing something with Dad, evoked tremendous affective responses from the mothers. The mothers' group leader was kept abreast of the assignments and was able to use this information to help the mothers express their feelings in their group. Sharing these experiences and helping each other through the pain was a very powerful aid to helping each group become cohesive and to experience each other's power to help through sharing similar histories and feelings.

Not every child in the co-terminus childrens' group had a parent in the mother's group. These members did not appear to suffer adverse effects because of this. For most of them, their mothers had previously been involved in a women's group. These children seemed to enjoy and derive a sense of satisfaction from the interactions of the two groups as much as the children whose mothers were in the group did.

We believe that a major missing link in building a comprehensive service for these children is the lack of services for fathers. Most violent men are themselves progeny of violent families. A group that deals with their issues as sons and fathers could clearly have significant impact.

CONCLUSION

The recognition that the children from violent homes constitute a population at risk is well documented by research. In-depth studies describe symptomatologies; social isolation, withdrawal, depression, aggression, fighting, and behavioural difficulties as being characteristic of many of these children. These studies have been instrumental in encouraging treatment services to meet the needs of this group of children.

Treatment for children from violent homes is still largely in the experimental stage. The primary service modality has been the peer group. While we concur with this choice we believe that models of service have not utilized social group work technology and, as a result, have neglected group process. In our experience with groups for these children, when processes are ignored, groups experience significant problems with behaviour, participation, and attendance, and have limited, often superficial, impact. When we attend to group processes and foster mutual aid in groups these problems diminish markedly and the children can make significant changes.

In the group they are able to more appropriately and directly express affect and to resolve nonviolently intra-group conflicts. Their sense of power to control their immediate environment seems to be increased greatly. What is more, reports from outside the group indicate that the children are applying their newly acquired skills and behaviours in outside contexts. These reports often cite improved peer interaction, improved behaviour at home and at school, improved academic performance, and improved family relationships.

While we hope that this paper has illustrated ways to foster the mutual aid process with this particular population, it is clear that more research and development are necessary. We believe that government and funding agencies and the agencies delivering services to the victims of domestic violence need to first recognize that the children in these families have service needs. The potential for group work intervention with this population needs to be exploited. The limitations of short-term, educational models of intervention must be confronted. The need for a longer term model that utilizes social group work technology and mutual aid must be recognized and supported.

NOTES

1. Giles-Sims, Jean, "A Longitudinal Study of Battered Children of Battered Wives," *Family Relations*, 1985, pp. 205-210. Hughes, H.M. and Barad, S.J., "Psychological Functioning of Children in a Battered Women's Shelter: A Preliminary Investigation," *American Journal of Orthopsychiatry*, 53, 1983, pp. 525-531. Sopp-Gibson, Susan, "Children from Violent Homes," *Journal of On-*

tario Association of Children's Aid Societies, 23 (10), 1980. Straus, M.A., Gelles, R.J., Steinmetz, S.K. *Behind Closed Doors: Violence in the American Family*, Garden City, N.Y., Anchor, 1980. Walker, L. *The Battered Woman*, N.Y., Harper & Row, 1979. Wolfe, D.A., Jaffe, P., Wilson, S. and Zak, L. "Children of Battered Women: The Relation of Child Behaviour to Family Violence and Maternal Stress," *Journal of Consulting and Clinical Psychology*, 53, 1985, pp. 657-665.

2. Rosenbaum, A. and O'Leary, K.D., "Children: The Unintended Victims of Marital Violence," *American Journal of Orthopsychiatry*, 51, 1981, pp. 692-699.

3. Jaffe, P., Wilson, S., Wolfe, D., and Zak L. "Family Violence and Child Adjustment: A Comparative Analysis of Girl's and Boy's Behavioural Symptoms," American Journal of Psychiatry, 143:1, Jan. 1986, pp. 74-77. Jaffe, P., Wolfe, D., Wilson, S., Slusczarzck, M. "Similarities in Behavior and Social Adjustment Among Child Victims and Witnesses to Family Violence." *American Journal of Orthopsychiatry*, 1985. Porter, B. and O'Leary, K.D., "Marital Discord and Childhood Behavior Problems," *Journal of Abnormal Child Psychology*, 8, 1980, pp. 287-295.

4. Garwood, S. *New Beginnings*, The Women's Interval Home of Sarnia-Lambton, Inc., 1985. Sinclair, D., *Understanding Wife Assault: A Training Model for Counsellors and Advocates*. Wilson, S., Cameron, S., Jaffe, P., Wolfe, D., *A Manual for a Group Program for Children Exposed to Wife Assault*, Unpublished, 1986.

5. Shulman, L. *The Skills of Helping Individuals and Groups*, Illinois, F.E. Peacock Publishers Inc., 1979.

6. Garwood, *op. cit.*

7. Shulman, *op. cit.*, p. 309.

8. Bion, William R., *Experiences in Groups*, N.Y., Basic Books, 1961.

9. Shulman, *op. cit.*

10. Sinclair, *op. cit.*

Feedback, Role Rehearsal, and Programming Enactments: Cycles in the Group's Middle Phase

Urania Glassman
Len Kates

The group–Sam, Gladys, Carl, Rhea, Sid, Rose, Paul and Wallace, as well as I (the worker) met outside the agency at 7 p.m. Thursday. Some members were car pooling in a van for disabled folks, others were in their families' cars. Wheel chairs, walkers, crutches, and other devices that support movement for people who are physically disabled could be seen. These young adults 18-21, were anxious and apprehensive about getting going to their first night out in the Ship Ahoy Single's Bar. I could see the smiles and grimaces as well as the tension on their faces. As recent victims of serious accidents–a year or two ago–they experienced depression and bitterness as well as fears of humiliation and embarrassment in their young adulthood. They all had dated and did no more; no place was set up for them; no one would easily accept them.

A sub-group and I had checked out the Ship Ahoy and figured there was significant access.

These parent-drivers, friends and siblings were anxious to help, to come too. The members made it clear once again, "only to the parking lot; then we get in ourselves no matter where the chips fall." Surprisingly, no one really looked up when we came through the door to a couple of round tables. It was dimly lit and noisy, but not yet full. People were rushing around. Sam said he knew a guy, Marvin, at the bar. Rose and Paul, now in wheel chairs, recollected dancing. Sodas, beers, chips are ordered. The members gawked, looked shy, talked to me, seemed to avoid contact with me. I chatted with all, keeping as real a conversational mood and tone as possible.

Gladys had to go to the rest room. She needed my assistance. Carl and I discerned it was empty. We crossed that bridge easily. What was astounding about the evening was that no one but the members really batted an eyelash at people who are disabled being there. During anticipatory role-playing the group had felt paranoid because the Ship Ahoy is such a "hot" singles bar.

Wallace and Sam got over near the bar, drinking and chatting. I got Rose with her walker onto the dance floor. We talked and laughed. The others looked around. A woman came over who knew Rhea and chatted with her. The manager, in a conspiratorial tone, asked me if they needed help. I said, "No, thanks, they are fine."

The group members were breathing easier, laughing, a little high. Conversation flowed, with a loss of awareness of the environment and people. They looked more into it and relaxed than I anticipated.

About 3 hours later, Sam's brother came in. He let us know the cars and vans were waiting. Members who were mobile left with each other. One by one, I wheeled others out. The tone and words were "See you at group next week."

INTRODUCTION

In this paper we will explicate a number of social group work techniques that appear in the middle phase as worker and members actively engage in actualizing the group's purpose. These are the techniques of programming, role rehearsal, feedback, confrontation, and group reflective consideration. They have been identified and described earlier, as 5 of 29 techniques of group work practice presented in our paper on the practice theory of group work technique (Glassman and Kates, 1986a).

We will return to this illustration of a group's program later on. If we were to immediately describe and illustrate each of the targeted techniques, we would be forgetful of the caveats in the earlier paper:

Many more steps beyond this exploratory work are needed . . . to shed . . . light on the . . . worker's use of self. . . . An in-depth examination of the use of each technique . . . would be illuminating. Further exploration of the use of techniques in the different stages of a group's development would be enlightening. (Glassman and Kates, 1986a, p. 37)

Thus, we will discuss the five techniques of group work practice, i.e., programming, role rehearsal, feedback, confrontation, and group reflective consideration, in the contexts of the objectives of group work method as well as group work stage theory. We feel that the frustration of immediate satisfaction of the urge for practical how-to-do-it approaches grows out of the imperative for knowing theory of technique. In this way one avoids mechanistic and unidimensional transactions between the group members and the worker.

PRACTICE THEORY ON TECHNIQUE: TECHNOLOGY AND ARTISTRY

The techniques of social group work have been defined earlier (Glassman and Kates, 1986a) as a set of specific behaviors the worker uses to help the social work group achieve its dual objectives–of developing a democratic mutual aid system and of actualizing the group's purpose. The specific techniques to be further discussed here (as is the case with all 29 techniques described in the earlier work) are used consciously by the worker in the life of the group as modes of professional self-expression in the process. Schwartz wrote the following about this state:

There is nothing in the conception of a professional methodology which denies or subordinates the uniquely personal and artistic component which each worker brings to the helping function. On the contrary, the concept of disciplined uniqueness is inherent in the definition of art itself. In a broad sense, we may view artistic activity as an attempt . . . to express strong personal feelings and aspirations through a disciplined use of . . . materials. (Schwartz, 1966, p. 29)

Schwartz helps us to recognize the interplay between disciplined uses of self and intuitive and emotional experiences. We have noted: "In the socioemotional processes among the worker and members, the worker more frequently uses techniques in intertwined rather than discrete forms. Only upon careful retrospective examination of the process can the techniques appear in more stylized and discrete forms" (Glassman and Kates, 1987, p. 7).

With these perspectives in mind, while one can conceive of a technique as a set of interrelated behaviors, the actual experience is a fluid one. (Our illustration of a group's program seems to bear out that impression.) The use of technique may be to a great extent the outcome of an interplay between the worker's intuitive processes and capacities for self-discipline in transaction with the group members' needs as they reflect the group's psychosocial purpose. Thus, while technique presented as codified aspects of behavior may introduce a worker to disciplined uses of self in the method, technique alone barely approximates the full panoply of group dynamics and nitty-gritty of human interaction experienced by the worker and members.

ON THE UNIQUENESS
OF THE SOCIAL WORK GROUP

The objectives of social group work differ from those of other professionally disciplined group methods. Social group work is a method of psychosocial problem solving which maintains and encourages the group as a social form (Lang, 1981; Glassman and Kates, 1986b). Worker activity in the social work group is geared to evolving a small group composed of people with similar psychosocial needs played out in natural and/or formal contexts. Papell and Rothman have indicated the social work group is characterized by ". . . common goals, mutual aid, and nonsynthentic experiences . . . where the group worker is directed to using the potential power which resides in the helping efforts of the members" (Papell and Rothman, 1981, p. 7). We have noted as well that the social work group, as part of the real life space of its members, can encompass members' use of social action for the enhancement of personal needs as well as their use of introspection to effect social change (Glassman and Kates, 1986a, p. 10).

On the other hand, if we look for a moment at traditional forms of group psychotherapy, the group as a social entity, i.e., its interpersonal life, is conceived to be secondary and more often is submerged in the interest of heightening transferential reactions which facilitate psychological interpretation of interpersonal phenomena (Glassman and Kates, 1983). This is not to say that some theories of group psychotherapy do not use group dynamics. Several do (Yalom, Stock and Whittaker especially), and have been relied on by social work clinicians interested in work with groups primarily because in these theories the group form is *not* fully submerged, thereby offering some consonance with social group work models. Also, in these models of group psychotherapy, there is less emphasis on transferential phenomenon and more concern with assisting members in achieving ego mastery in their current contexts. In such a group there is some examination of the group's interpersonal life as a replica of members' patterns of relating. Still, the traditional psychotherapy group, while using some of the egalitarian participatory processes that engender mutuality, is focused on the relationships as *means* towards achieving psychological ends. In fact, the relationships built in the group are not encouraged to flourish but are disallowed beyond the group in the interest of maintaining a sociological neutrality. In another group form–the T-group, the small group as a social form is not only maintained, it is heightened and scrutinized as well. The raison d'être of the T-group is its development solely for the purpose of studying its dynamics–its structures, norms, leadership patterns, and authority relations. There is no other psychosocial purpose beyond this self-study.

The social work group uniquely represents characteristics of the T-group and psychotherapy group in its social milieu. It shares with the T-group its attention to the formation of a participatory, just, and caring group, grounded in democratic norms and decision making processes; this is an important goal (not unlike the concerns of Kurt Lewin, the father of the T-group). The social work group is conducted by a nonauthoritarian worker who challenges the group members to review their approach to and relationship with authority. Social group work shares with group psychotherapy the goal of individual change and growth; it translates these interests into role enhancement or through functional experiences in and out of the group. Social learning and role enhancement in the social work group optimally occur in a context of democratic perspectives and interaction. Furthermore, in the social work group, change also occurs in relationships among members beyond the group meeting time itself. This externality (Papell and Rothman, 1981) reflects the centrality of the social environment in social group work method. Therefore, developing humane and democratic group forms within the context of the social milieu while enhancing significant social role relationships is uppermost in the development of a group work practice theory of technique. The worker and the group are engaged in an interactional venture for creating alternatives in social living. All have a stake in the process; growth and role enhancement are germaine for the members; professional role enhancement is germaine for the worker (Glassman and Kates, 1987).

PRACTICE THEORY FOR ACHIEVING THE SOCIAL WORK GROUP AS A UNIQUE ENTITY

The Dual Objectives

Lang (1981) has noted that in the social work group the development of democratic norms is central. These norms are the means of interaction that guide patterns of group development. Lang has noted that democratic norms need to evolve somewhat before group members are encouraged to actively work on achieving their psychosocial objectives. Taking off from Lang's seminal work, we feel that there are two distinct yet interrelated objectives in the social work group. These are the development of the democratic mutual aid system and the actualization of purpose. (See Glassman and Kates, 1986a, 1986b; Lang, 1981, p. 24; Papell and Rothman, 1981.) The development of the democratic mutual aid system and the actualization of purpose guide the mutual efforts of the social worker and group members throughout group life. The social worker first focuses on enabling the members to evolve expansive ways of interacting, while subduing members' self-motivated urges to intensely work on psychosocial theme-centered issues. How we are working on our goals is a significant group question. This is so for several reasons. Members have yet to develop ways of working with each other. Members need to take time to examine how they are relating to the worker's authority, how they have interacted in previous authority situations, and how they are dealing with the need to develop group norms. Still, members will go through naturally and methodologically stimulated stages of development and change in their capacities to interact; these will require substantial and inclusive behavioral norms. In addition, the working-on and working-through processes for actualizing purposeful change require commitment, as well as a high degree of affective connection between the members and the worker. Particular kinds of interactions among members help the development of the Democratic Mutual Aid System. These are:

Forms of Interaction that Foster the Democratic Mutual Aid System

- Developing and appreciating democratic norms, which include rights to belong and to be heard.
- Making decisions and developing rules.
- Developing leadership and followership skills.
- Respecting differences amongst members.
- Expressing feelings about the worker with particular attention to authority issues.
- Collectively developing and setting goals.
- Expressing feelings towards members.
- Developing affective bonds and furthering cohesion.

As the members come to value and make use of democratic humanistic norms (Glassman and Kates, 1986b, pp. 148-167) they move more effectively towards the second objective of actualizing group purpose. Here, difficult agendas for change are undertaken; the nature of the interactional processes is altered; and more frequent processes of interaction that foster the group's purpose are in evidence. These are:

Forms of Interaction that Foster the Actualization
of Purpose

- Identifying themes to be worked on.
- Expressing role enhancing behaviors.
- Expressing and identifying feelings that help the group and members work on change.
- Sharing perceptions and feelings about each other's behavior.
- Creating activities in the milieu.
- Identifying group process issues and structures to heighten the group's self-awareness.
- Identifying projections and self-fulfilling prophesies as they interfere with collaboration and role-enhancement.
- Reflecting on and reinforcing individual and group change in order to replicate change.

As these interactions manifest, practice theory and clinical experience assume that the members and worker become increasingly engaged in a broad spectrum of interactions. These interactions relate to the members' purposes both in, as well as out of, the group's meeting environment. Members take on a variety of tasks at different levels of satisfaction and difficulty. Some issues and tasks might seem insurmountable to members. It is rarely easy and simple to give up dysfunctional behavioral patterns in the interest of enhanced role performance. Yet, it is in the caring, supportive and productive environment of the democratic/humanistic group that each member finds the ways and means to work-on and work-through real life experiential processes in the group and out of the group.

The Dual Objectives and Stage Theory

Interactions for actualizing purpose occur within stages of a social work group's development (Garland, Jones and Kolodny, 1973; Glassman and Kates, 1983). In terms of stage theory, when members have sufficiently worked out the authority and control issues they have a more expansive range of democratic interpersonal norms. With these they move in consistent ways into processes for working on purpose. The members including the worker have moved from the first and second stages of Pre-Affiliation and Power and Control, into the third and fourth stages of Intimacy and Differentiation (Garland, Jones and Kolodny, 1973). (In generic terms, the group has moved from beginning into the working-on and working-through processes of the middle phase.)

During the Intimacy and Differentiation Stages, but most particularly during the Differentiation stage, member behaviors are more consistently connected and apparent to one another. The worker's behavior is more apparent and open to members' scrutiny as well, not so much in transferential terms, but in regard to the worker's professional role behavior (Glassman and Kates, 1987). In an earlier paper we identified two themes related to the view of the worker during the Differentiation period. One was, "We're O.K. and Able" and the other was "This Isn't Good Anymore." As the group members are able to realistically accept both themselves and the worker, flexible cohesion and an expansive role repertoire develop. At the same time, increased motivation and capacity for change are highlighted. Obstacles in the change process may place the group into a fight mode which leads to denigrating members' abilities and prior achievements. This fight mode, fleeting in some groups, pronounced in others, needs to be dealt with empathically and nonjudgmentally rather than defensively. (See Glassman and Kates, 1983.) All in all the worker in the Differentiation Stage examines his/her own process of expression and is called upon to be emotionally mature, unguarded, and engaged to serve as a role model for the members' participation and reflectiveness (Glassman and Kates, 1987).

Techniques Used to Achieve the Dual Objectives

The worker uses specific practice techniques to help the group master the interactions that center on developing the democratic mutual aid system and actualizing group purpose. Techniques have been identified, specified, and categorized in terms of their primary uses in helping the group meet these objectives (Glassman and Kates, 1986a). Some techniques were found to be used by the worker throughout all stages of the group's development.[1] Some techniques are used primarily to develop the democratic mutual aid system.[2] Still others are used primarily to actualize the group's psychosocial purpose. These are: data and facts, role rehearsal, programming, group reflective consideration, dealing with the unknown, feedback, conflict resolution, self-disclosure, interpretation, group mending, and taking stock.

At this point in the paper, with the establishment of the methodological context, programming, feedback, role rehearsal, confrontation, and group reflective consideration will be examined. We will discuss their use and application, returning to examine our opening illustration for a better understanding of the relationship of these techniques to one another in the group's interpersonal life as members work on actualizing purpose.

THE USE OF TECHNIQUE
TO ACTUALIZE PURPOSE

It is through disciplined uses of self that the social worker expresses techniques. The working-on and working-through activities of the group constitute its efforts to actualize its purpose or its raison d'être. These activities enable members to become more effective in their roles in the actual milieu designated by the group's psychosocial purpose.

The Relationship Among Techniques for Actualizing Purpose

Practice experience indicates that worker's use of programming, role rehearsal, feedback, confrontation, and group reflective consideration, occur in some type of relationship to one another as the participants center their efforts towards actualizing their purpose. If we define member self-expression as social interaction, ideas, attitudes, feelings, moods, fantasies, and physical activities, we note that only the worker's use of programming stimulates the possibility for members to experience the full range of role expression. The other techniques do not usually include full forms of interaction and physical activities. In addition, if we look at the milieus in which the members often carry out the effects of these techniques, i.e., the meeting itself, and/or the members' social environments outside of the group, we note that programming occurs in both of these. In fact, programming should probably occur more frequently in the external milieu rather than in the meeting itself, to encourage and support real-life experiences rather than replications. The other techniques (role rehearsal, feedback, confrontation, and group reflective consideration), are probably more often used by the worker within the group's meeting environment.

It appears that there is a difference in kind between programming and the other techniques. Interactions and experiences encouraged by programming stimulate the use of the other techniques.

PROGRAMMING

In social group work, the worker uses techniques of engagement to motivate action and other forms of interpersonal expression to motivate behavioral change. Programming stimulates a panoply of experiences and interactions among the group members and with significant others in their external and group environments. Programming is facilitated by worker activities through interrelating steps in the process. Steps in programming are: (1) *Initiation.* The worker initiates the members to goals and means of programming, indicating that its derivative experiences offers them opportunity to change and develop new skills and capacities; (2) *Discussing options.* The worker stimulates discussions of alternative program scenarios, focusing on the relationship of these to members' needs; (3) *Tasks and Tools.* The worker encourages the members to identify situations, tasks, and approaches, and to secure materials; (4) *Program execution.* The worker is actively involved, providing support, sharing in the experience, serving as a role model, and protecting members' security; (5) *Evaluation.* The worker engages the members in rehashing the experience; they consider how it fulfilled the members needs, its high points, its low points, and implications for future options.

Programming, a technique encompassing several worker behaviors, stimulates the group's "externality," one of the distinguishing features of the social work group (Papell and Rothman, 1981). To meet its goals the group needs to develop programs in the actual social environment–often for all the members, sometimes for some, and sometimes inclusive of significant others in the members' real lives. The worker relinquishes varying degrees of control by sharing in the program while not being necessarily bound to participate in the actual program. The worker appropriately moves to the background as the primary social and emotional connection to members (Glassman and Kates, 1987). However, whether or not the worker is present during the program, the result of the worker's efforts and disciplined approaches ought to be evidenced by the members.

Of the five steps in Programming, Step 4, Program Execution, is of a different kind and quality. It is the result of a disciplined process involving the worker in helping the group organize its collective resources towards purposeful action. The last step, "Evaluation," is a propellant for additional program ventures.

The psychosocial events in the programming process represent a full range of behavioral transactions among members, complementary others, and unanticipated others, in the group's or members' natural and/or formal milieus. The total programming process focuses on and reflects the actual experiences that bring the members together. Programming is experienced within the values of the democratic humanistic social work group. For the members, the psychosocial program is a proving and improving ground. Programming is a means to help members be reflective in meeting their own needs as well as those of significant others. In this vein, a social work group's psychosocial programs (stimulated by the worker using the steps in the technique of programming), are the most significant statements of what makes this professionally guided group a social work one. The program reveals and brings to life the group's objectives and goals.

The young adult group's night in the singles' bar illustrates a program execution. It was partially the result of the worker's use of "initiation," "discussion of options," and "tasks and tools" in a partly directed, off the cuff, yet professionally guided process. It had started five weeks earlier when members grumbled and cried that they could not go out again. The worker had said that was " . . . a bunch of bull . . . ," and later motivated a commitment to go out. By using the steps in the worker technique of programming, the worker did not give the members a chance to ruminate their way out of it.

One key aspect of programming is its flow with the organic psychosocial needs and interactions of group members. The technique, programming, appears clearly and systematically ordered to remind the worker of necessary business. It is not ordered to lock the worker or group into a fixed agenda and process. In fact, programming could start with a rather seemingly spontaneous happening. Then the program event can generate more orderly and planful programs.

The experience of the young adults who were disabled led to some especially poignant sessions following the program. These sessions were rather unpredictable too, because each meeting really is an existential entity unto itself. And, as well, an actual program experience stimulates new feelings, desires, awarenesses and directions for the members.

GROUP REFLECTIVE CONSIDERATION

This worker technique (described as an important case work one by Hollis, 1972, pp. 125-138) is used in group also, to help members look at recent past experiences that relate to the group's purpose. As a re-focusing tool it can lead to new ideas, attitudes and perceptions. The worker asks members to recall the aspects, contexts, and affects of particular experiences. Attention is paid to the sequencing of events, feelings and interactions to re-enliven and reconstruct the behaviors and feelings. Effort is made to keep the discussion focused on detail rather than muddied generalities. The worker then asks the members how these awarenesses are affecting them right now (Glassman and Kates, 1986a).

Motivating and moving this process not only generates its desired behavioral forms, it also brings into scrutiny and exposes for all to see, attitudes, feelings, perceptions, desires and agendas that members have. Furthermore, the forms of cooperation and inclusive communication test the metal of the group as a democratic mutual aid system, giving the members another chance to accept and modify this fabric of special norms (Glassman and Kates, 1986b).

Thus, the worker also finds her/himself using "processing the here-and-now," a technique used more often in the formation phase to institutionalize intergroup relations and strengthen the formation of democratic norms. This technique actively involves the members in the immediate examination of the group's behaviors primarily to foster ownership of the "how-we-are-and-will-be" of the group as an entity. The worker periodically asks the members to identify the group's salient events as the dynamics are unfolding (Glassman and Kates, 1986a).

Illustration of Group Reflective Consideration

The group reconvened Thursday. The worker as usual met people in the parking lot, down the ramp and into the room. People nodded and breathed sighs of relief about last Thursday's event at the Ship Ahoy. When all were in the room, I drew them into a kind of circle and said, "We'll do well to go over the events and experiences we all had last Thursday." Rose just burst out crying. All of us, including myself, were totally shocked. Her father had scolded her about thinking she would be able to "really" go out. He said this in the car going home. The members comforted her, literally and figuratively wiping her tears. Others spoke of actual and impressionistic feelings that their relatives were not supportive. Rose repeatedly said no one would help her pee like I helped. The mood and tone were "poor me," "victim," earmarked by talk about their relatives. I said, "Look at what is happening right now; what's the interaction?" Wallace astutely said "We're all just like we were when our relatives first dropped us off." Rhea said, "Were there changes? I don't feel like I felt around the table Thursday. I was horny and hot to trot." Carl chimed in that the group should pull itself together and kick that dad's butt by bringing him to the Ship Ahoy ". . . next time we go." The flow of interaction moved back to what happened and what will happen ". . . if we go again."

FEEDBACK AND CONFRONTATION

"Feedback" and "confrontation" are two other techniques effected in the differentiation processes of the group's life. Feedback is used by the worker to help members give individuated responses in the context of an interdependent system. Feedback helps members clarify feelings they have about each other and their behaviors. When receiving feedback, the member learns how others are reacting to his/her behavior, while at the same time coming to recognize that not everyone is affected in the same way by experiences and behavior. The worker may begin the process by encouraging members to share from the "I perceive and I feel" perspective, modeling for the members how to proceed.

Confrontation is used sparingly by the worker in the middle phase of group life to help members face patterns of activity and attitude that are dysfunctional, painful, and divisive. Confrontation is used to help members to change in the group context along with other members. Both feedback and confrontation are marked by direct expression of feelings. However, feedback is characterized by tact, perception, and some efforts towards consensual validation, whereas confrontation is marked by directness, strong feelings and behavioral change. Both connect to actual here-and-now experiences. Confrontation aims to change a pattern; feedback helps the members gain perspective.

The group program provides vital experiences and opportunity for members-in-role to work-on-and-through their needs and interests.

Illustration of Feedback and Confrontation

During the program evaluation, Carl looked to Rose and used feedback. He said, "When you cry like you just did, it makes me see you as completely dependent; I think you feel lost." (I realized that the group members had incorporated the use of feedback in their interactional repertoire.) Others too gave feedback to Rose. She was rather relaxed and composed, being both a bit curious and skeptical about Carl's perceptions. She guessed she just triggered his softheartedness, and was busy with "I like it too because deep down I feel O.K. about going out again." Carl started taking back his perceptions and feelings. "Stop it Carl," I said. "Turn toward Rose; control yourself and tell her directly what you are thinking and feeling about what she said just now." Carl turned pale, lifted his face, looked at Rose, and said aloud, "Bull, you aren't sure you can deal with your father about going out. And others of us–me too, aren't sure about it also." (He looked directly at everyone.) He continued, "I heard people say they were scared shitless and their relatives avoided talking with them." I said, "No better time than to set up for another night-on-the-town at the Ship Ahoy, three Thursdays from tonight . . ."

ROLE REHEARSAL

Role rehearsal goes hand-in-hand with programming. Programming brings group members into the real world; It requires preparation. Role rehearsal brings members in touch with their potential capacities to change in situations with others. In using role rehearsal, the worker engages the members in imagining and sharing feelings and actions they anticipate. The worker helps by focusing the group towards detail in order to develop strategies and options that enhance their role repertoires beyond their habituated patterns. A further step may involve "formalized role play" in which the worker and group develop the role play situation from the needs of the members encouraging them to try out new forms of expression (Glassman and Kates, 1986a).

Illustration of Role Rehearsal

After deciding to return to the Ship Ahoy, the group went back to talking about reactions of their relatives. Carl said that his mother worries about him all the time, and that while he wants to get a driver's license, she is reluctant and afraid. Rhea said that it sounded like her father. He "worries about me and maybe he's just being overprotective when he says I shouldn't go out. "Sam said he had already talked with his brother about these things. Others seemed to feel it was a big issue. I asked Sam to tell the group what he had said to his brother. He said "I told him that though I get depressed and lose heart a lot, I want him not to feel sorry for me or to think that I can't do it. I told him that I needed him to give me strength." Carl began to cry, saying that he wanted to say these things to his mother but was afraid to. I suggested he tell us how he would approach her. He said he would tell her he needed to have his driver's license and a car with hand brakes. I asked him what he thought she would say. He anticipated she would offer to drive him herself. I asked Carol to "Go on, what would you say." Rose spontaneously moved in front of Carl, "Make believe I'm your mother, talk to me." After thinking, he said, "Ma, I can't go on depending on you; I can learn to drive again. And I *can* become strong enough to put the chair into the car. I know guys going to the gym using the machines to build their upper bodies." I asked him to tell us how he felt right now saying these things to his mother. He said he felt braver, like he could do it. The group seemed to feel more relaxed from this. I asked other members to talk about how they would approach their loved ones. After more discussion, the group then went on to talk about how they wanted to go out to other places but were afraid. Sam said he used to like rock concerts but feels there is no way he can go to them anymore. Further discussion, anticipation of obstacles and role playing occurred . . .

THE CHANGE PROCESS

The practice theory of technique and the real life processes of the worker and group point to some type of cyclical relationship among the use and effects of techniques. The change process in the group involves a continuous cycle of trust, risk and experimentation with new behavior. The cycle begins with less formed early steps in the trust, risk, and experimentation continuum. It results in successes and failures in the members' attempts to master change. The change cycle gains momentum by further repetitions of the continuum. As work progresses, more complete states in the trust, risk, and experimentation cycle are effected creating a series of forward movements which represent a spiral of change. The worker intervenes in this process by using techniques to help members effect change. Thus, a spiral-like process occurs between worker behavior as technique, and member behavior as experience. This spiral represents and encompasses the working-on and working-through effort in the group (Glassman and Kates, 1987).

For the group of disabled young adults, mastery of the role and life-style changes, as well as the range of feelings and attitudes of loss, anger, resentment, and futility, in combination with hope and further attempts to explore options, will not be an easy process. The members will stumble, literally and figuratively, as they continue to find new ways to prop themselves up in order to engage life and project themselves into the future.

As noted previously, the program execution itself, as an apparent part of the chain of events, is of a different order and kind for the member, in that it is an experience in the member's real life. For the worker, the programming technique encompasses the broadest use of self and offers the widest opportunity for experiencing and expanding each member's capacities. In generating these many chances for member mastery and growth, this technique encompasses the other techniques of role rehearsal, group reflective consideration, feedback, and confrontation.

CONCLUSION

We have examined the interrelationship among five important techniques of group work practice used primarily to effect change in the middle phase of group life, and have explored their interplay when applied to the practice reality. We have found that when conceptualizing technique, a central issue for the practitioner is to keep the flow going *always* in the direction of the group's experience. The worker is thereby challenged to use these interrelated techniques consciously–with a keen eye on the creative spiral of interaction–in order to effect spontaneous and empathic uses.

Obviously, we are stimulated towards further examination of the relationship among some of the other techniques we have identified in our earlier work, as they are illustrated in the live group. For instance, the techniques of "processing the here-and-now," "collective participation," "inviting reactions to the worker role" and "decision making," which have such an important effect on group formation, deserve further study. In addition, systematic research needs to be undertaken as well that sheds light on the worker's use of techniques during the entirety of a group's life.

REFERENCE NOTES

1. Some techniques used in all stages include the more generic social work techniques of lending a vision, demand for work, exploration, identification, staying with feelings, silence, directing, confrontation, and support.

2. Some techniques used primarily to develop the democratic mutual aid system are: facilitating collective participation, scanning, engaging the group as a whole, modulating the expression of feeling, facilitating decision making processes, processing the here and now, expressing feelings about the worker role, goal identification, and good and welfare.

REFERENCES

Bennis, Warren and Shepard, Herbert A. "A Theory of Group Development," in Warren Bennis, Kenneth Benne and Robert Chin (Eds.), *The Planning of Change*. N.Y.: Holt, Rinehart and Winston, 1962, pp. 321-340.

Boyd, Neva. "Social Group Work: A Definition with a Methodological Note." Paul Simon (Ed.), *Play and Game Theory in Group Work: A Collection of Papers by Neva Boyd*. Chicago, Ill.: The Jane Addams Grad. School Social Work, 1971, pp. 141-154.

Falck, Hans, "The Membership Model of Social Work," *Social Work* 29:2, 1984.

Garland, James A., Jones, Hubert A. and Kolodny, Ralph, "A Model for Stages of Development in Social Work Groups" in Saul Bernstein (Ed.), *Explorations in Group Work: Essays in Theory and Practice*. Boston: Milford House, 1973, pp. 17-71.

Glassman, Urania and Kates, Len. "Authority Themes and Worker Group Transactions: Additional Dimensions to the Stages of Group Development," *Social Work with Groups* 6:2, Summer 1983, pp. 33-52.

Glassman, Urania and Kates, Len. "Techniques of Social Group Work: A Framework for Practice." *Social Work with Groups* 9:1, Spring 1986a, pp. 9-38.

Glassman, Urania and Kates, Len. "Developing the Democratic Humanistic Norms of the Social Work Group," in Marvin Parnes, (Ed.), *Innovations in Social Group Work,* N.Y.: The Haworth Press, Inc., 1986b, pp. 149-167.

Glassman, Urania and Kates, Len. "On Actualizing Purpose in the Social Work Group: Approaches to the Middle Phase." Paper presented at Symposium for the Advancement of Social Work with Groups, Boston: October 1987.

Hollis, Florence, *Casework: A Psychosocial Therapy.* N.Y.: Random House, 1972.

Klein, Alan. *Social Work Through Group Process.* N.Y.: SUNY, Albany, 1970.

Lang, Norma C. "A Broad Range Model of Practice in Social Work with Groups," *Social Service Review* 46:1, March 1972, pp. 76-89.

Lang, Norma C. "Some Defining Characteristics of the Social Work Group: Unique Social Form," in Sonia Leib Abels and Paul Abels, (Eds.), *Social Work with Groups: Proceedings 1979 Symposium,* Louisville, KY: CASWG 1981, pp. 18-50.

Levine, Baruch, *Group Psychotherapy, Practice and Development.* Englewood Cliffs, N.J.: Prentice Hall, 1979.

Middleman, Ruth R. *The Non-Verbal Method in Working with Groups.* N.Y.: Association Press, 1968, reissued, Hebron, CT: Practitioners Press, 1981.

National Training Laboratory Participants Manual, 1966 and 1967.

Papell, Catherine P. and Rothman, Beulah, "Social Group Work Models: Possession and Heritage," in Albert Alissi, (Ed.), *Perspectives on Social Group Work Practice,* N.Y.: The Free Press, 1980.

Papell, Catherine P. and Rothman, Beulah, "Relating the Mainstream Model of Social Work with Groups to Group Psychotherapy and the Structured Group Approach," *Social Work with Groups* 3:2, 1981.

Schwartz, William, "Between Client and System: The Mediating Function," in Robert W. Roberts and Helen Northen, *Theories of Social Work with Groups,* N.Y.: Columbia University Press, 1976.

Schwartz, William, "The Social Worker in the Group" in Ruby B. Pernell and Beatrice Saunders, *New Perspectives on Services to Groups: Theory, Organization and Practice,* N.Y.: NASW, 1961, pp. 17-28.

Seitz, Martin, "The Issue of Membership in the Social Work Group." Paper presented at the CASWG Symposium, 1985.

Shulman, Lawrence, *The Skills of Helping Individuals and Groups,* 2nd ed. Itasca, Ill.: Peacock Press, 1984.

Vinter, Robert, "An Approach to Group Work Practice," in Paul Glasser, Rosemary Sarri, and Robert Vinter, *Individual Change Through Small Groups,* N.Y.: The Free Press, 1974.

Whittaker, James K. "Models of Group Development" in Albert Alissi (Ed.), *Perspectives on Social Group Work Practice.* N.Y.: The Free Press, 1980, pp. 135-153.

Yalom, Irvin D. *The Theory and Practice of Group Psychotherapy.* N.Y.: Basic Books, 1975.

Small Group Dynamics
and a Dialectic Discourse

Salvatore Imbrogno

INTRODUCTION

Social work often draws distinctions between the perceptions of "ideal ends" in macro-practice and the conceptions of "real world" micro-practice. These role distinctions in practice have a detrimental effect on the actual and potential contribution of social group work to policy analysis and development. As one way to avoid this pitfall, this paper examines the dynamics to the following interconnecting problems: (1) What is the integrative role of small group policy bodies in the seemingly dichotomous process of macro-level policy formulation and micro-level policy implementation? (2) How can small group policy bodies interrelate social group work policy theory with the dynamics of small group practice?

Therefore, the primary focus for analysis rests in a twofold design: (1) to create a unified conceptual framework of critical theory from which the methods and processes of a dialectic discourse are derived for applications to social group work; and (2) to demonstrate the primary role that social group work methods and skills have in social policy development (Checkoway, 1986).

A dialectic discourse is a principal method for the expression of critical theory in practice. It refers to". . . a situation of absolutely uncoerced and unlimited discussion"; a process that leads to emancipation and enlightenment (Guess, 1981, p. 65). A dialectic discourse entails a social group process that strives to achieve optimal conditions for rational decision making. Optimal conditions refer to an environment in which "non-deprivation, non-coercion and minimally correct information" prevails (ibid., p. 52). This process leads to a rational consensus of the real and true value and interest of the affected constituents.

A first task is to describe and analyze these basic principles of critical theory within the context of diametrically opposing positions: contradictory, competing and conflicting values of small groups involved in policy development. Models for confronting opposition are presented with an eye toward the dynamics of group work processes. Intrinsic to this task is the application of critical theory towards converging macro-micro level professional social group work practice (Cnaan and Adar, 1987).

Finally, competing paradigms for social group work policy bodies are presented to explicate the differences between mainstream and emerging group work activities. Social group work methods and procedures for the initiation, design and implementation of a dialectic discourse and a rational consensus are presented.

SMALL GROUP POLICY BODIES
AND CRITICAL THEORY

Similarities in conceptual perspectives exist between professional social group workers and critical theorists. Both seek to achieve a unity between what is conceived conceptually and what must be put into action. Both are concerned about the conflicting and contradictory claims made by groups representing different values, interest and belief systems on policy. A plurality of group attitudes, behavior and motivations necessary for taking policy actions have generated a number of different intervention modalities.

For example, one means for resolving differences is for social group workers to adopt a broker's role in connecting a group or community system with needed resources (Connaway and Gentry, 1988). Social group work has a long history, beginning with the settlement house movement, serving as an advocate in securing, protecting and promoting the human and social rights of an affected constituency. Social group work activities provide opportunities for learning social skills to improve individual and group role performance. Creating innovative social and community programs have always been part of a professional group worker's arsenal.

These mainstream intervention modalities generally perceive opposing values, interests and belief systems as falling within the purview of mediating problems and conflicts between parties and arriving at social adjustments. In a policy context, the social group worker's role is identified as a facilitator. In direct contrast, a critical theory perspective views an expression of diametrically opposing positions as providing an arena for small groups to contribute to a meaningful dialogue for social change. The social group worker's role is to create an open, noncoercive environment in which opposing and competing values on a policy issue, problem or conflict can be freely expressed. A new intervention modality is being introduced to augment rather than replace mainstream group work policy practice.

The dynamics of social group processes when placed within the context of a dialectic discourse, connects the ideals of policy formulation (i.e., what does it mean?) with the realities of implementation (i.e., how will it work?) in one social setting. No restrictions, limitations or omissions can be placed on information in an open dialogue between small group policy bodies. For example, information is equally accessible to those involved in prospective analysis of goal formulation at a board meeting and for those involved in executing a social program, activity or service in a social agency.

Positions taken by groups on opposing values generally represent a slice of a preconceived reality. Interest groups formulate their common ends based on a parochial conception and specification of policy. Policy actions are taken through idiosyncratic methods. Taken together they create an ideological position with hypothetical boundaries for negotiation. A dialectic discourse seeks to reconcile competitive paradigms by building into the inquiry a broader paradigm. This reduces or eliminates parochial perspectives and in so doing, provides opportunity for complementation. As a result, opposing groups are theoretically unified and free to reach higher levels of inquiry and discourse (Sutherland, 1978).

Critical theory and the processes of a dialectic discourse are value laden. A primary value commitment is to human dignity and emancipation. An important way to realize this is through free and open communication between groups of different values, interests and belief systems (Benhabib, 1986). A thoughtful expression of differences, a reasonable challenge to those with opposing positions and or clarity in the presentation and interpretation of different values are critical attributes to human and social growth and development. This view of group dynamics envisions the potential for a rational consensus: an optimal condition for social change in which all parties are beneficiaries.

As noted, social group work as a function in policy practice emphasizes mediation and facilitation to resolve differences primarily through compromise and bargaining. A dialectic discourse is an alternative modality for intervention. It builds on differences as a means to achieve a more advanced and higher level of understanding. For example, mediation of value dilemmas and facilitating resolution through a "community of minds" is a viable, expedient and a pragmatic mode of intervention (Churchman, 1971). However, it leads to social adjustments and not change. Melioration is a strategic move away from a social problem and not problem solving.

A dialectic discourse, on the other hand, compels small groups to change their parochial positions through argumentation and confrontation. As noted, a competitive dialectic discourse moves to produce change through policy problem solving. This inevitably raises the level of inquiry to a higher level of abstraction. A dialectic discourse is not only the most parsimonious and constructive way by which to benefit from the dynamics of group processes but it is the only meaningful way to grow and develop under adversarial conditions.

THE INNATE AMBIGUITY
AND INDETERMINACY OF POLICY

What precipitating factors create opposition and ambiguity as critical factors in all stages of the policy process?

At least four principles provide a reasonable explanation:

1. A social policy will produce changes in existing social and behavioral group processes. Social policy is expected therefore, to generate stress, strain and tension in individuals and small groups in organized life.
2. Individual and small group perceptions and expectations of policy are often incongruent with those making policy and the agency itself.

3. Policy must be formulated to be sufficiently flexible to become operational. The meaning of policy evolves from the various interpretations given by those affected by it. Managers are expected to take discretionary actions to make an "ideal" operational.
4. The policy process impacts on the stability and the adaptive mechanisms set in place by groups in organizations. This generates new structural patterns and relations between members and across systems. Structural and behavioral changes in group relations is a primary reason for resistance, opposition and obstacles to policy implementation in social agencies (Rein, 1970).

In sum, a social policy process accompanied by its intrinsic qualities of ambiguity and indeterminacy when juxtaposed to the multiple values and interests of stakeholders, generates an environment of continuous conflicting and contradictory claims on policy (Brockriede and Ehninger, 1960).

MODELS OF CONFRONTING
DIAMETRICALLY OPPOSING POSITIONS

A number of conceptual models suggest modes of intervention for small group work practice.

Separation

The critical components that comprise human and social content, processes and outcomes in policy can be separated analytically to provide causal explanations for variations on values, interest and belief systems. There is great reliance on the transferable value of natural and physical laws of "scientism" to draw distinctions through reductionism of the components that comprise social phenomena.

A logical and rational analysis can explicate different positions taken on a continuum of extremes (i.e., fact/value, right/wrong, quantitative/qualitative, objectivity/subjectivity; truth/falsity). In terms of human and social factors, choices can be conveniently made in an "either/or" position. For example, a social problem of homelessness is one of technological know-how in the mobilization, organization and management of resources. Or a policy problem of homelessness can be viewed as one of conflicting, contradictory and antagonistic ideologies intrinsic to a system that created the condition in the first place.

Given an "either/or" choice offers an avenue for avoidance of confrontation or argumentation through adopting feelings of alienation or by strategically withdrawing into isolation.

Separation by physical distinctions in social and human roles and functions reflects a top/down, unilateral decision making and deterministic policy model. For example, small group policy bodies consist of top level executives responsible for policy formulation. They are separated from those on line whose daily practice decisions are expected to comply with policy. The latter are viewed as thinkers; the former as doers. Social work group practice in well-structured settings (i.e., closed systems such as the military, mental institutions and prisons) are particularly subject to these structural distinctions.

Oppressor and Oppressed

Opposition can be viewed as the inevitable by-product of hierarchical levels of authoritative relations in social agencies where one rules (i.e., elite) and all others are ruled. Compliance and submission is achieved through use of power. Power and not conflict is the independent variable. Power in this context is defined as a self-imposed elimination of choice in acting upon someone else's orders. An organizational structure and its control mechanisms govern the conditions under which individuals and small groups are given license to determine the meaning given to policy. This negates the use of ingenuity and spontaneity associated with the dynamics of small group processes.

The oppressor and the oppressed produce a bifurcation model for behavioral relations towards opposition. Social agency executives are given authority and acquire exclusive power over policy formulation, social processes for implementation and informational networks of an agency. The "tyranny of the group" inevitably arises to create a social agency organizational structure that determines the who, when, where, how of small group performance and participation in policy. Often the oppressed replace the oppressors and in turn, themselves become tyrants.

Conflict

A struggle exists between the enhancement, maintenance and preservation of existing values representing the advocates of policy (status quo) and alternative values representing an adversary group. The latter are standing by in opposition waiting to replace those in power. Polar opposites when taken to an irreconcilable state necessitate a discontinuance with each position in a move towards a more advanced conflict conception of a problem solving model. More specifically, problems are solved between competing groups over the short run pending the inevitable emergence of intermediary problems and conflicts. This briefly characterizes a revolutionary interpretation of social change over the long run.

This is a classical view of the dialectic: one position reflects the maintenance and preservation of a social agency's existing policy (thesis) while another group is advancing major changes in purpose and direction (antithesis). The only way out of the dilemma is a synthesis that encompasses past values (thesis) with present expectations (antithesis) to create a new policy for the future.

Diametrically opposing positions characterized by this interpretation of the dialectic takes contradictions as highly antagonistic and irreconcilable. When compounded by the notion of discontinuity as the only basis for change, conflict produces the fruits for coercion and a potential for violence. (This stands in direct contrast to a dialectic discourse as advanced in this paper.)

A social agency must be prepared to function under conditions of short-term stability. It must be designed to discontinue existing social norms and values periodically for new and different sets. Conflict produces a trifurcation of behavioral relations in the same social agency: small groups advocating the existing values of the agency, small groups resisting by offering alternatives while a third is responding in new and broader perspectives to agency policy.

Social group work methods in social and community action never fully adopted a Marxist view of the dialectic for social change. For example, social group workers seldom advocated purposive exacerbation of a conflict situation as a means to produce major social change.

Harmony

A major distinction needs to be drawn between a classical interpretation of dialectic materialism (i.e., antagonistic and irreconcilable positions generated by conflicts in social and materialistic conditions for distinctive positions) and the approach taken in this paper of a dialectic discourse (i.e., open, uncoerced environment of argumentation and confrontation of differences as a means to achieve mutually interdependent positions). The attributes of a classical interpretation of a dialectic discourse are placed within the harmonious conception of opposing values.

Opposition in policy is seen as concurrently a bipolar complementarity and as mutually inclusive. For example, and as noted, small group policy bodies formulate goals and objectives while small groups in various programs and services execute policy. These are usually designated as distinct organizational functions. Yet, while top level policy is determining lower level decisions the consequences of these decisions are impacting on the purpose and direction of policy. There is a mutual exchange of information "in and about" policy from a top/down and bottom/up interactive process. If it is accepted that values are intermittently introduced in the process, then policy is indeed dynamic, continuously changing and in a state of flux.

Hence, values, roles and functions of participants in a harmonious conception are continuously interacting to produce changes in organizational design, policy formulation and implementation. By grasping the dynamics of a multiplicity of group activity, an innovative social group work function is to grasp the dynamics of a multiplicity of group activity (i.e., a reciprocity of small groups) and integrate them into a collectivity that ensures stability under changing conditions. An underlying expectation of a "holistic" perspective is to produce new challenges and directions for policy development.

Changes in small group practice results from a continuous interaction of contrasting and similar forces for creative growth and self-maintenance. New knowledge and information is produced in the process of formulating and executing policy. The result is changes in policy and in the organizational design of an agency. For example, a social agency should be effecting external changes in the community in which it functions. External changes are fed back into the agency as new value inputs changing the purpose, function and direction of the agency. It is reasonable to expect social workers and their groups to enhance and elevate their problem-solving capabilities as a result of this process.

In sum, in the real world of human and social group interaction, an integration of different values, interests and belief systems results in complementary patterns of opposites: separation and integration, convergence and divergence, love and hate. The choice taken on any one position for conceptualizing opposition reflects upon the kinds and types of methods chosen for social group work practice. We are selecting an harmonious complementation of opposing values as the foundation upon which to build a unified conceptual framework for the integration of dialectics into social group work policy practice. My intent now is to explicate the attributes of harmony and the methods of congruency for "confronting opposition" as the most viable and parsimonious method for social group work in macro-practice.

EMERGING ROLE OF THE SOCIAL GROUP WORKER IN MACRO-PRACTICE

A number of key observations can be established from this analysis that requires a fresh look at the role and function of group work in social policy development:

1. Individuals, small groups and the worker in search for an optimal position in a maze of a multiplicity of values and a diversity of interest, must view policy as both a determinant of lower level decisions (independent variable) as well as a consequence of these decisions (dependent variable). A number of lower level decisions in aggregate result in the real meaning given to policy. Social group

workers must be familiar with the dynamics of all stages to policy development in formulation (macro), transformation (mezzo) and implementation (micro), preferably from an ecological perspective.

2. Opposition is ubiquitous to the multi-levels of the policy process: policy planning and development, program planning and management, and project planning and operations (Mayer, 1985). Social group workers must further develop their methods and skills to "treat" adversarial, conflicting and opposing positions as a natural and desirable state of policy development.

3. A social group worker must view each stage of policy as an actual or potential source of conflict and contradictory claims on policy. However, through the use of group dynamics and methods of a dialectic discourse, a group worker can integrate the functions of each stage and their corresponding value systems to arrive at more efficient decision making and more effective policy performance.

In sum, the social group worker must view all stages and multi-levels of social policy development as a critical arena for professional macro-practice. A dialectic discourse offers an opportunity to integrate the various components to policy through a rational consensus. A key objective is to coalesce different values through a process that increases the level of policy activity and performance of all affected constituents.

INTEGRATION OF CRITICAL THEORY, RATIONAL CONSENSUS AND SOCIAL GROUP WORK

Critical theory provides a conceptual framework by which the professional can initiate a social group process designed to purposefully provide parties holding opposing positions the opportunity to present, defend and justify their policy claims in all stages and levels of policy development. It is important to emphasize that a social agency must be designed to ensure individual and group access to all stages so as to generate a horizontal and vertical exchange of information. It is only through the use of small group dynamics, within the context of this conception, that all affected constituents can genuinely engage and reach a higher and more harmonious level of collective behavior.

Let us examine four principles derived from critical theory that govern the conditions for small group policy bodies:

1. Conditions can prevail that are not coercive and where information is made available and subject to scrutiny by all participants (Guess, 1981). One critical role for the professional social group worker is to help create a free and open process in a climate of meaningful and positive discourse resulting in conflict resolution. Secondly, a key to effective social group work practice lies in the acquisition, utilization and sharing of appropriate information by all affected constituents.

2. Creating optimal conditions for a rational consensus is a formidable problem. An optimal condition implies "perfect knowledge" about solving a policy problem (i.e., varying desirable ends are both known and agreed upon). As noted, there exist a plurality of values many of which are in disagreement, unknown, diffused and/or unacceptable to some elements in the community. Social group workers have an educational role in enabling affected constituents to develop the practical research skills to organize, formulate and present their positions. This helps to unravel the complexities of opposing positions. It also serves as an important way to establish "perfect knowledge" or identify the obstacles and hindrances leading to an optimal condition. Group work as a social and rational process is a practical way to achieve rational consensus.

3. Hence, critical theory focuses on what is a rational process. More specifically, under what conditions can a policy process become a rational one? Striving for optimal conditions is not an utopian exercise. A dialectic discourse is a social process in which free communication is viewed as an ideal way in which to abolish some of the coercion and intimidation from which groups suffer. Needless to say, an important asset is that it enables groups to move closer to an optimal condition and "perfect knowledge." This can be designated as a social work group heuristic function in providing a framework to enable groups to make their next moves.

4. A search for the optimal conditions is realized through a comprehensive and unified policy process. Different values and interests are explicated for rational consensus. Social group workers in

this context strive for optimality as a focal point in which to integrate idiosyncratic perspectives and parochial positions. Hence, a social group worker actively observes and participates in a group process of synthesis; an optimal form of creative rationality.

In sum, the thrust of this theory is to advance the idea that truth can be derived from a rational consensus. A rational consensus can only be explicated in a social process that identifies and defines the strategies, tactics and modes of argumentation through which it can be derived at (Benhabib, 1986, p. 288).

A PARADIGM FOR INCREMENTAL AND RATIONAL CONSENSUS

Let us now examine, within a decision making context, two major paradigms to social group work policy practice. Each accepts value dilemmas as the basis for decision making. Each responds to conflicting and contradictory values in different ways. Obviously emphasis will be placed on the emerging role a dialectic discourse plays in social group work dynamics.

As noted, the mainstream social group work paradigm advocates mediating conflictual positions through compromise and bargaining. An incremental consensus ("small change") is realized when opposing positions (i.e., those making a demand on the norms and values of the system) agree to concede some elements of their values and interests for conflict resolution and consequently, also agree in process to preserve and maintain the system's basic values and norms.

Each problem presented is an original perturbation to the existing value system. It is also noted from the onset that problems will not be solved but resolved in a move away from a social ill. "Muddling through" is not a purposeful planned change model. In contrast to a rational consensus, alternative courses of action and their consequences must be marginal and dependent upon existing policy values. This is the essence of incremental consensus.

Value inputs as a course of action must "fit into" the patterns and relations of the system. Preceding decisions are treated as fragmentary entitles. They serve to remedy a social perturbation and to integrate each value input into the existing value system. As a result, the original configuration of the presenting problem changes with the preceding adjustments of the means/ends to a problem. (Braybrooke and Lindblom, 1962).

In contrast, rational consensus is not reactive, meliorative, expedient or necessarily pragmatic. Rational consensus refers to an interactive developmental process absolutely uncoerced and where unlimited discussion between "free and equal human agents in unconstrained dialogue prevails" (Guess, 1981, p. 65). In this context too, a unity of opposition differs from utilitarian aspects of social adjustment. "Greatest happiness for the greatest number" in a community of interest and social adjustment does not necessarily bring about just ends. Those on the extreme are eliminated in this concept of social utility.

Rational consensus is not engineered to be pragmatic in the sense of achieving expediency, forming coalitions or to mitigate a problematic situation over the short run. Practicality in rational consensus is to show the way. Additionally, it is very much different from the use of coalitions to influence social policy (Gentry, 1987). Coalition formations, like many other modes of intervention presented, adapt an incremental/pluralistic conception of "mirroring the past."

A concept of equal and unconstrained dialogue eliminates the either/or distinctions expressed in oppressor/oppressed and conflict relations which characterized the nature and quality of confronting opposition. Entering into a group's interactive process for the sole purpose of satisfying idiosyncratic values and parochial interests is eliminated. The optimization of any one value is contingent upon the optimal conditions that are created by the contribution and participation of a collectivity in a dialectic dialogue. A rational consensus model serves as its own system control.

METHODS AND PROCEDURES
FOR A DIALECTIC DISCOURSE

It is now propitious to enumerate upon the basic conditions under which a rational consensus process can be put into use by the social group worker so that the various modes of argumentation (i.e., advocacy claims) and motivations for individual and small group participation, contributions and commitment can be activated in all three stages and multi-levels of policy development.

1. Each participant and small group acting as a collectivity must be given equal opportunity to impact on a dialectic structure by participating in the setting of an agenda for argumentation; share in determining a course and direction for deliberations; a length of time for communication and to be informed on who are the participating parties.

2. Each participant (and small group) must be open for confrontation in the raising of questions; demanding justifications for claims made and providing explanations within the context of a discourse.

3. All participants must be given equal opportunity to express their needs, interests, desires and expectation without any internal or external constraints on discourse. A climate must be created where participants know that they will be heard. It is assumed that an open and free discourse encourages a social interactive process of a genuine and honest exchange of information.

4. Individuals and small groups must have equal access to information particularly where it is known that conflicting and contradictory claims will emerge in response to a policy issue or problem. This ensures equal chance to make assertions, recommendations, provide explanations and to challenge others in a confrontational but thoughtful manner. No one is exempt from questioning and criticism. This minimizes domination (i.e., mobilization of a bias) while encouraging others to be accountable for their behavior (Bachrach and Boratz, 1970).

5. All participants know that they play a major role in determining the purpose and direction of the policy process and that the norms built in by social agency structure do not become policy ends in and of themselves.

These conditions set the stage for rational consensus that goes beyond analytical distinctions which strive for mediation and lead to mediocrity. A rational consensus includes a process of creative synthesis in a unification of opposites. This conceptual framework deliberately sets a stage for elevating a discourse to a higher level of complexity (i.e., more enlightened criticism, emancipation and reflection); and ensures social agency and community growth and development, while simultaneously maintaining stability under changing conditions.

CONCLUSION

This paper examined distinctions drawn between theory and action, which if not confronted in a dialectic discourse, are designed to reflect and reinforce the status quo of existing small groups of power elites. Social phenomena, especially in macro practices, are permeated with a multiplicity of values and a diversity of interests, elements of which are chosen by individuals and small groups as policy claims. Critical theory produces a method to achieve a rational consensus as an alternative to mainstream modes for intervention. Stages of policy development and multi-levels of structural complexity were examined in relation to the dynamics of a reciprocity of individuals in small groups and a system integration in a reciprocity of small groups in a collectivity. These processes were introduced as cognitive and motivational factors for individuals and small groups to pursue optimal conditions for a rational consensus. Conditions for establishing a dialectic discourse and for realizing a rational consensus were enumerated for application to social group work practice on a macro-micro level.

REFERENCES

Bachrach, P. & Baratz, S. (1970). *Power and Poverty: Theory and Practice.* New York: Oxford University Press.

Benhabib, S. (1986). *Critique, Norm and Utopias: A Study of the Foundation of Critical Theory.* New York: Plenum Press.

Braybrooke, D. & Lindblom, C. (1963). *A Strategy of Decision.* New York: The Free Press.

Brockriede, W. & Ehninger, D. (1960). Toulmin on Argument: An Interpretation and Application. *The Quarterly Journal of Speech.* 46.

Checkoway, B. (1986). *Strategic Perspectives on Planning Practice.* Lexington, Mass: Lexington Books.

Churchman, C.W. (1971). *The Design of Inquiring Systems: Basic Concepts of Systems and Organizations.* New York: Basic Books.

Cnaan, Ram & Hadasa Adar. (1987). "An Integrative Model for Group Work in Community Organization Practice." *Social Work with Groups.* Vol. 10, No. 3, Fall.

Cox, F., Erlich, J., Rothman, J. & Tropman, J. (1987). *Strategies of Community Organizations.* Itasca, Il.: F.E. Peacock.

Gentry, Martha. (1987). "Coalition Formation and Processes. *Social Work with Groups.* Vol. 10, No. 3, Fall.

Gilbert, N. & Specht, H. 2nd. Ed. (1986). Dimensions of Social Welfare Policy. Englewood Cliffs, N.J.: Prentice Hall.

Grinnel, R. (1981). Social Work Research and Evaluation. Itasca, Il.: F.E. Peacock.

Guess, R. (1981). *The Idea of a Critical Theory: Habermas and the Frankfurt School.* London: Cambridge University Press.

Kettner, P., Daley, J., & Nicols, A. (1985). *Initiating Change in Organizations and Communities.* Monterey, CA.: Brooks/Cole.

Mayer, R. (1985). *Policy and Program Planning: A Developmental Perspective.* Englewood Cliffs, N.J.: Prentice Hall.

Mayer, R. & Greenwood, E. (1980). *The Design of Social Policy Research.* Englewood, Cliffs, N.J.: Prentice Hall.

Piece, D. (1984). *Policy for the Social Work Practitioner.* New York: Longman.

Rein, M. (1970). *Social Policy: Issues of Choice and Change.* New York: Random House.

Sutherland, John. (1978). *Societal Systems: Methodology, Modeling and Management.* New York: North-Holland.

Not Just One of the Gang:
Group Workers and Their Role
as an Authority

Roselle Kurland
Robert Salmon

Students of group work often have negative attitudes toward authority and are uncomfortable with the idea of themselves in positions of authority. It is the authors' contention that many are attracted to group work because they believe mistakenly that in a group, democratic participation and a spirit of equality will magically occur from the very start and they will be able to sit back and participate as "one of the gang." Students may view their exertion of authority as synonymous with imposing their ideas onto group members, something they wish to avoid at all costs. As a consequence, group workers often do not provide the structure and direction that groups and individual group members need, especially in the early stages of group development.[1] What often follows the group worker's abdication of his/her role of authority are groups that fall apart prematurely and unnecessarily.

Three related areas regarding the use of authority will be discussed in this paper. They are:

- student attitudes toward authority and toward themselves in positions of authority;
- methods and techniques and critical times that can be used by social work teachers and supervisors to help students develop greater awareness of and comfort in the use of the authority inherent in their roles;
- the central impact of teachers and supervisors as persons in positions of authority in serving as role models for students.

BACKGROUND

Authority may be defined as a power delegated to the practitioner by client and agency in which the practitioner is seen as having the power to influence or persuade resulting from possession of certain knowledge and experience and from occupying a certain position. Thus there are two aspects of authority in the helping relationship. The first might be called the institutional aspect in that it comes from the social workers' position and function within the agency's purpose and program. The second aspect is psychological in that clients give workers the power to influence or persuade because they accept them as sources of information and advice–as experts in their field.[2]

It should be understood that being an authority, in a position of power, often has been an issue for social workers, and not only social group work students. Goldstein commented:

. . . it has been the tendency of social workers to disclaim the role of authority and the idea that any degree of power was used in practice. Equality, cooperation, and the recognition of others' rights were valued precepts; any manifestation of power and control would therefore be seen as the antithesis of these principles and as an abuse or manipulation of others' rights.[3]

Even those in our profession who have achieved legitimated positions of authority with inherent power, may experience difficulty with the authority aspect of their role. Authority and power may be equated with authoritarianism, and viewed with distaste, and denial of its legitimacy. "The predominant view of power . . . is much like the Victorian view of sex. It is seen as vulgar, as a sign of character defect, as something an upstanding professional would not be interested in, stoop to engage in."[4] To this point, Alfred Kadushin, in *Supervision in Social Work*, cited research which repeatedly showed social work supervisors failing to use their authority and power in implementing the responsibilities of the supervisory function.[5] The verbal commitment to the values of democracy and autonomy often obscure or overlook the fact that *all* helping relationships essentially involve influence and authority.[6] Many contributors to the literature have helped us to recognize this.[7]

Helen Northen, in discussing social workers' actions with their groups pointed out that workers who deny the fact that they have authority also may not recognize or accept the concomitant responsibility for the welfare of the group. In the desire to be liked as a friend, they confuse democracy and laissez-faire leadership, sometimes abdicating their role, or becoming authoritarian as ways of handling their feelings. This is bound to provoke severe testing by the group members who expect the worker to give professional opinions and take appropriate action in the group.[8] Students, in particular, may not understand that the workers' acceptance of the responsibilities of their authority role provides clients–the group members–with a sense of security and safety.

> A person in need of help seeks someone who has the authority of knowledge and skill to be of help . . . The attempt of social workers to abdicate their role and pretend that they carry no authority only leaves clients troubled by suspicions and doubts about why workers are unwilling to admit what they, the clients, are so aware of.[9]

Despite the references to the literature, already cited, the difficulty that social workers may have in exercising appropriate authority with their groups, and the negative results of this problem, have not been given a great deal of attention. It is not that concerns about authority are absent from the social work literature about groups. However, much of the material deals with the group's need to work out authority issues with the worker, rather than with the worker's need to develop comfort and skill in exercising his/her role of authority.

Social work theorists have given great attention to group members' struggles with authority. As examples, the Garland, Jones and Kolodny model consists of five stages of development with its major focus on the socio-emotional issues facing the group members. The second stage, Power and Control, includes rebellion against the group leader as one of the basic issues to be coped with, and resolved.[10] William Schwartz, in his interactionist approach, describes Authority and Intimacy as the two main themes that characterize the group members' way of working together. In the theme of Authority, the group is occupied with their relationship to the helping person, and the ways in which this relationship is instrumental to their purpose.[11]

The importance of the "authority" and "intimacy" themes owe much to group dynamics literature, particularly the work of Bennis and Shepard.[12] However, there is wide acceptance in the social group work literature that these two central constructs have meaning for all groups.[13] Also, there is agreement that the authority theme will be paramount in the beginnings of group development. Shulman makes this point, as follows:

> . . . Group members have to deal early in The Life of the Group, with their relationship to the leader–the authority theme. Many of the central issues have to do with dependency; that is, how dependent will the group members be on the leader.[14]

However, the worker's need to deal with his/her own authority in relation to the group is of great importance, for group life and group survival, and this aspect has not been given equal attention. Shulman commented, "One of the most difficult feelings a supervisor must come to grips with is the role of the outsider."[15] This applies to workers and students who lead groups as well and it is the fact that the leader, the authority figure, is "not one of the gang" that makes it so difficult. Group work instructors, in the way they teach, serve as role models for the students, and they can help enormously by demonstrating effective use of their authority with the class group.

STUDENT ATTITUDES AND STRUGGLES

A survey of 25 students majoring in group work conducted at the end of their first year of MSW study indicates that struggle with their role as an authority was characteristic of their first-year experience.

Four major interwoven concerns of students contributed to their struggle: (1) a desire to be liked and accepted by the members of the groups with which they worked; (2) lack of clarity about the social work role and about what it means to be in a role of authority; (3) fear that they did not possess the knowledge and skills necessary to assume the role of worker with a group; and (4) fear that group members would react negatively to their assumption of a role of authority.

Student responses on a questionnaire asking them to describe their attitudes toward and experiences with authority illustrate these four concerns. Looking back at his first-year experience, one student said, "I don't like being in authoritative positions, telling other people what to do. I'd much rather be part of the group, given direction instead of providing it. It's much easier. You don't have to think as much and it's safer because people won't tell you that you're wrong. It's a fear of rejection." The desire to be liked and accepted was echoed by another student, "Looking back, I walked into the group feeling as if I were a member in it, not a leader. I was so preoccupied with being liked and accepted that I lost sight of my role."

Lack of clarity about role and questioning of ability is underscored by another student, "At the beginning of the school year, I didn't understand what being in a position of authority entailed. Although I knew the leader was to be a facilitator, I felt uncomfortable with being in a position of authority. I asked myself why I was there and there were internal voices that doubted my qualification." Another student stated, "I felt apprehensive, afraid I didn't have the skills, afraid I wouldn't be able to maintain control or make intelligent decisions."

Concern that group members did not want the worker to assume a role of authority and would react negatively to his/her doing so was expressed by another student. "I wanted to see myself as more of a peer in the group–one of the gang. I thought if the group saw me as an authority they wouldn't feel comfortable opening up." Said another student, "I worried that members would project past negative experiences with authority figures on to me and would resent and dislike me."

Being a student seemed to add to the uncertainty that was felt about their role as an authority as did differences in age and race between students and their clients. "As a student, how much authority did I have?" asked one student. "How much could I act independently of my supervisor even when/if I wanted to? I struggled with that." Another student, in her mid-20s, who was asked to supervise activity leaders, many of whom were older than she, in an after-school program for latency-age children underscored age as compounding her struggle with her role as an authority. "I usually consider people who are older than me to also be wiser, even when they might not be as experienced in a particular area. I sometimes feel like a kid when I have to supervise or confront people older than I am. That definitely happened this year."

For another student, who worked with a group composed of Black and Hispanic men in a temporary shelter for the homeless, differences in race and class contributed to the difficulties he experienced with authority. "I am uncomfortable about being white and middle class. Although I probably make too much of my discomfort over these aspects of myself, I still feel uncomfortable. How do my clients view me? I see that as an obstacle and because of that I hold back."

By the end of their first year of graduate study, students reported that they had become more comfortable assuming a role of authority. The actual experience of working with groups and the increased skill that such work with groups brought about as well as the enhanced understanding of groups and group process that resulted from both class and field experiences increased students' confidence and willingness to exert their authority.

Students credited the actual experience of working with groups with helping them to better understand how to be and use their authority. Said one student, "Now I feel more confident in a position of authority because I have seen some success in the groups I have worked with. As I experience more group work, I'm coming to understand how authority should be 'worn'." Another student also linked experience with increasing confidence and noted, "I'm becoming more confident–that's the most important factor. If you feel confident, others will pick it up and feel confident too. Then authority is not as threatening."

The link between increased skill, gained from class and field, and increased confidence, comfort, and willingness to exert authority was emphasized. Said one student, "I feel more confident about the way I'm handling myself now. I have more skill and I feel more effective than I did at the beginning of the year which helps me to be more comfortable in assuming authority." Said another, "Learning that I *do* have some knowledge and skill and also that I don't have to be perfect and have all the right answers, that I can admit when I make a mistake–these things have led me to be more comfortable in a position of authority." Another student also emphasized the importance of increased skill. "I think my initial ambivalence about being in a position of authority had more to do with not knowing what to do than it had to do with egalitarian values . . . I struggled with the acquisition of techniques and knowledge to use authority effectively and not co-opt it from the group . . . As I've learned how to function more skillfully as a leader, I'm finding that being in a position of authority is ceasing to be an issue."

Finally, increased understanding of and knowledge about groups and group process were important in increasing students' willingness to assume their authority. Said one student, "I'm more able to accept a position of authority for myself now because I have more confidence in the process of group work. That makes me feel less that I am responsible for all that goes on in the group. Because of that, I'm more comfortable." Another student noted, "I realize that I don't need to be the one who's 'on top' in order to be in position of authority."

Some students seemed surprised at the demand by the members of the groups with which they worked that they assume a role of authority. "Whether I like it or not," said one, "my groups treat me as an authority figure." Similarly, another student commented, "My groups treated me as an authority in their lives, even when at first I did not want to be." Still another student said, "I realize now that it isn't really possible *not* to assume a role of authority. In fact, I've come to think of it as an abuse of authority if the leader *doesn't* assume a role of authority. You can either be an authority figure who is passive or one who actively assumes the role, but you'll still be one no matter what. If you are aware of assuming the role, your interactions are more thoughtful." Another student, working with teens in a high school setting, commented, "I've grown more comfortable as an authority figure through noticing that the group really seems to *need* me in that role. It seems to be a very good experience for them to have a positive, constructive interaction with an authority figure. If you abdicate that role, they don't have this opportunity."

TEACHING OPPORTUNITIES

The subject of authority, especially the new worker's discomfort with a role of authority, needs to be addressed directly in group work practice classes and in supervision in the field. Especially at the start of class or field work, when students are struggling with defining the social work role, opportunities abound to ask them to consider their own attitudes toward authority and toward themselves in positions of authority.

Above all, three questions promote such discussion and help students grapple with their attitudes toward and view of themselves in positions of authority:

1. Think about persons in positions of authority with whom you have worked in the past. Identify those you think carried out their authority role either very well or very poorly. What was characteristic of the way in which they did so? And what are the implications of that for your own social work practice with groups?
2. What are some of the fearful fantasies you have as you envision yourself in your first meeting with a group? What do you envision as some of the worst things that might happen?
3. What *do* you have to offer to clients with whom you work, especially clients who are different from you in significant ways, such as age, race, and/or experiences?

Discussion that results from these questions provides an opportunity to begin to address the concerns of students about authority identified earlier. Asking students to look at others in positions of authority helps them look at the social work role and what it means to be in a role of authority. Asking them to identify what they have to offer to clients different from themselves helps them identify the knowledge and skills that they possess and/or want and need to develop. Finally, asking students about some of the fears they envision helps them first voice and then discuss the negative ways in which they fear group members will react to them along with their desire to be liked and accepted by group members. That question usually opens up the subject of control in the group, what control means, what it actually "looks like" in group work practice. Through discussion of that, students can be helped to grapple with their often simultaneous desires and tendencies to be overly controlling on the one hand and overly passive on the other.

Nowhere are the students' tendencies to be too passive more apparent than in the beginning stage of group development and nowhere are the students' tendencies to be too controlling more apparent than in the work phase.[16] Thus, the beginning stage and the work phase in group development are two teaching areas in both class and field that are crucial in providing opportunities to help students learn about and develop greater comfort with their role of authority.

In the beginning stage of group development, members' ambivalence, anxieties, wariness, and fears call for the worker to be active in providing direction and structure for the group and its individual members. Yet most new students, in beginning their work with a group, express a strong desire to not impose upon or dictate to the group. They want the group to truly belong to its members. Students do not want to exert their authority at this time. They shy away from providing leadership because they fear that to do so is synonymous with imposing upon the group and will detract from the members' active participation and ownership of the group. Thus, the needs of group members in the beginning stage, for direction and structure from the worker, and the priority as seen by student workers, to not impose upon the group and its members, are often contradictory.

That contradiction between member needs and student priorities in regard to the worker's role of authority needs to be highlighted for class discussion. The following excerpt from a first-year group work class is an example of one way in which such a contradiction may be expressed and can then be examined.

Barry reported that he had met for the first time with a boys group consisting of eighth graders who were having academic and social difficulties in the Junior High School they attended. He said they had spent a lot of time during the first meeting deciding on group rules and he thought it had gone well because the boys had participated pretty actively and everyone had voted for the rules the boys made up. But now he didn't know what to do because the boys had made up some pretty strict rules and he didn't know how he was going to enforce them. They all voted that there was to be no cursing and the rule was that if you cursed three times in one meeting you'd have to leave the group for that day. They also decided that if someone had to leave two group meetings because they'd been cursing, then they were out of the group altogether and couldn't return to future meetings.

"I think that if they don't like the group, then some of the boys will get themselves thrown out on purpose," Barry said. "And I also think it's unrealistic to think there won't be cursing in the group," he added.

Class members agreed that Barry was in an untenable position now, since he'd be spending a lot of time enforcing a rule that didn't make sense and that it was not unlikely that cursing would become the center of the group's attention in a way that was not necessary and that would not be helpful to the group.

Discussion centered on Barry's role in the rule-making process. He admitted that he had sat back a lot and let the boys make the rules on their own, even when he realized that the rules they were making up were going to be problematic. "They were actively participating and I didn't want to take away from that," he said. "If I had objected to the rules they were making up, I was afraid they'd clam up and let me dictate to them like their teachers do in class. I wanted them to see that this group was different from a class and that I was going to be different from a teacher."

Class discussion then centered on how Barry might have handled the rule-making process differently and how he might express some of the doubts he had voiced in the group work class directly to the group at its next meeting.

Once this student's specific dilemma was addressed, discussion could then take place around ways in which other students in the class had similarly not provided enough direction in the beginning stages in the groups with which they were working. Many specific examples were cited by students. The contradiction between members' needs and student priorities in regard to authority was identified as a theme common to beginnings.

During the work phase of the group it is not uncommon for students to be overly controlling in their use of authority. By assuming sole responsibility to "solve" the problems that arise in the group, by taking everything onto their shoulders alone, students unwittingly ignore the group and deprive the group and its members of opportunities to learn, grow, and develop. At this point in the life of the group, students need to understand that being in a position of authority does *not* mean doing everything *for* the group and having all the answers. Instead, the ability to observe what is taking place, to share one's observations honestly with the group, and to make a demand for work by asking the group to address the issues and problems that arise are crucial aspects of group leadership and the use of one's authority.

The following example from a first-year group work class highlights this aspect of the worker's role and use of authority.

> Mary said that she was having a lot of difficulty with her group, composed of elderly members in an agency that serves the blind. The group had two factions that were not getting along. One faction consisted of white members who tended to talk a lot and dominate the meetings. The other faction consisted of black members who were fairly quiet during the meetings. The two sub-groups did not mix. They sat on opposite sides of the room and did not talk to each other. Sometimes when one of the white members was talking, Mary said she noticed that some of the black members whispered to each other and didn't seem to be listening. Mary said she'd asked them not to whisper when someone was speaking, but that didn't seem to help very long. She'd also tried to draw in some of the black members by calling on them directly, but that had not worked well either.

Mary said that she thought the difficulty was being caused by the racial differences among the members. She said she did not know what to do and wondered whether anyone in the class knew of exercises she might use to get the two subgroups to mix more. "If I don't figure out something to do, I'm afraid the black members are just going to stop coming," she said.

In the class discussion that followed, the student's tendency to take responsibility from the group was identified and acknowledged. The need for her to share directly with the group her observations about what was taking place was pointed out. Other students were able to identify times when they had acted similarly, taking everything onto their shoulders and thereby becoming overly controlling in their authority by not confronting the group with and asking group members to work on difficulties they observed.

TEACHERS AS ROLE MODELS

Some of social work students' most important learning about authority comes from their observations of the ways in which their teachers behave. Students look to teachers and supervisors as important role models. How teachers carry out their own authority–what they actually do–may be even more important than what they teach about authority.

McKeachie identifies six distinct roles[17] which, in reality are components that are crucial to the teachers' overall role as an authority.

- First, teachers are experts. In this role, they transmit information, concepts and ideas.
- Second, teachers are formal authorities. They represent the school, setting goals and the procedures for reaching them, including the establishment of structure, assignments, standards of excellence and evaluation. Since students ascribe legitimacy to the authority of teachers, it is within the teachers' power to define what is relevant for class discussion, who shall speak

in class, and what kinds of classroom behavior are acceptable or unacceptably disruptive.

- Third, teachers are socializing agents, representing the profession, and through their own behavior, clarifying expectations and acceptable behavior.
- Fourth, teachers are facilitators. They help students define their own goals, encourage their creativity and independence, and work with them to enable them to reach their goals. Teachers must be good listeners, able to bring students out by helping them identify and sharpen their own interests and skills, insightfulness, and problem-solving capacities.
- Fifth, teachers are ego ideals. They convey their enthusiasm and excitement, as well as enjoyment of their subject, and of teaching. Crucial to teachers in this role are their energy, self-confidence, and ability to communicate that their subject is valuable and deeply important.
- Sixth, the teacher is a person. Teachers want to be validated by their students as human beings within the relationships that develop in the classroom. Students, in turn, have a similar need for validation. To achieve such validation, teachers reveal aspects of their personal selves as they teach and try to communicate that they are trustworthy and warm enough to encourage students to be open as well.

Social work students' descriptions of positive role models indicate that the components of the authority role that McKeachie identifies are of critical importance. The role components of expert, facilitator, and ego ideal were given special emphasis and importance by the students in describing positive authority figures. Students were clear that their positive attitude was related to people in authority who possessed knowledge, expertise and enthusiasm for their work, conveyed respect for others, and encouraged quality work and the active participation of others.

One student cited a former teacher as a positive role model. "She had very clear expectations and was even a little demanding. She enjoyed working with students and was excited about her work. She had a lot of confidence about her own work and worked very hard. She was generous about sharing her thoughts and was accepting of different points of view." Another student described a former dance teacher, "She spoke with absolute confidence in her instructions but always listened to others as if she was learning things that were more important than she taught."

Describing a former supervisor, one student said, "She led a group with a strong presence but always to the end of getting the widest possible participation from everyone present. She was interested in the group's ideas and feedback." Another student, also describing a supervisor, noted, "She made me *think* and figure things out for myself. She had a nice balance. She was easygoing, flexible, reasonable, yet she demanded satisfactory work. She welcomed input from others, yet was secure and confident about what she knew."

The students' analyses indicated that they were careful observers of their teachers and often tried to incorporate positive aspects of what they saw into their own styles of work. What students can learn through observing their teachers is directly related to the difficulties students have in carrying out their role of authority in the beginning and work phases of group development.

Considering how skilled teachers of group work began with their classes often helped students move past the passivity of their own beginnings with their groups. Experiencing the teacher making demands of the student for increased skill and commitment as the class moved on, often would be translated into their own practice as they would try to help clients do more for themselves, rather than doing the tasks for the clients.

Since the students will, to some extent, model themselves after the teachers they respect, perhaps one of the most important characteristics for the teacher is that of passion–passion for the subject, and learning, to be connected to the work with the clients. Another is the ability of teachers to acknowledge their own mistakes. When teachers do this, they send a clear message about their own humanity and professional fallibility. When students see that teachers can acknowledge mistakes, correct them, yet maintain appropriate control, it is a source of relief for them. They may understand that they too, can accept and learn from their own mistakes, without losing control.

CONCLUDING STATEMENT

Issues about authority are discussed frequently in the group work literature. But that literature tends to examine the struggle of group members in relation to authority. Discussion of the struggle of the group-leader in maintaining an appropriate authority role is limited. For students and new workers, accepting themselves as authority figures is crucial to their effectiveness as practitioners.

Teachers and supervisors need to be sensitive to and aware that the practice problems that students encounter frequently have as an underlying theme the students' difficulties in assuming a role of authority. They need to bring forward for explicit discussion this basic practice issue. In addition, teachers and supervisors need to be conscious of their own behavior in serving as some of the most important authorities and professional role models for their students.

NOTES

1. See, for example, material on the beginning stages of group development in James Garland, Hubert Jones, and Ralph Kolodny, "A Model for Stages of Development in Social Work Groups," in Saul Bernstein, ed., *Explorations in Group Work*, 1965; Helen Northen, *Social Work With Groups*, 1988, Columbia University Press; and Lawrence Shulman, *The Skills of Helping Individuals and Groups*, 1979, The Peacock Press.

2. Beulah Compton and Burt Galaway, *Social Work Processes*, The Dorsey Press, 1984, p. 204. Alfred Kadushin, in *Supervision in Social Work*, Columbia University Press: New York, 1985, p. 87, indicated that authority needs to be distinguished from power. Authority is a right which legitimates and sanctions the use of power. It is the right to issue directives, exercise control, require compliance, to determine the behavior of others, to make decisions which guide the actions of others, etc. On the other hand, power is the ability to implement the rights of authority.

3. Howard Goldstein, *Social Work Practice: A Unitary Approach*, University of South Carolina Press, 1973, p. 83.

4. Daniel Levinson and Gerald Klerman, "The Clinician-Executive Revisited," *Administration in Mental Health*, 1972, Volume 6, pp. 53-67.

5. Alfred Kadushin, op. cit., p. 103-107.

6. Max Siporin, *Introduction to Social Work Practice*, New York: Macmillan Publishing Co., 1975, p. 294.

7. As examples, see: Elliot Studt, "An Outline for Study of Social Authority Factors in Casework," *Social Casework*, 1954, 35: pp. 231-238, and "Worker-

Client Authority Relationships in Social Work," *Social Work*, 1959, 4 (1): pp. 18-28. Also, see Robert D. Vinter, "The Essential Components of Social Group Work Practice," in Robert D. Vinter, (ed.), *Readings in Group Work Practice* (Ann Arbor: Campus Publishers, 1967), pp. 8-38.

8. Helen Northen, op. cit., p. 226.

9. Beulah Compton and Burt Galaway, op. cit., p. 240.

10. James Garland, Hubert Jones, and Ralph Kolodny, Op. Cit.

11. William Schwartz, "On the Use of Groups in Social Work Practice," in William Schwartz and Serapio Zalba, (eds.), *The Practice of Group Work*, New York: Columbia University Press, 1971, p. 9. For a discussion of this theme, as it evolved in practice see Benjamin Stempler, "A Group Work Approach to Family Group Treatment," in Albert Alissi, (ed.), *Perspectives on Social Group Work Practice*, New York: The Free Press, 1980, pp. 310-325.

12. Warren Bennis and Herbert Shepard, "A Theory of Group Development," *Human Relations*, 1948. Vol. 9, pp. 415-37.

13. Alex Gitterman and Lawrence Shulman, *Mutual Aid Groups and The Life Cycle*, F.E. Peacock Publishers, Itasca, Illinois: 1986, p. 43.

14. Ibid.

15. Lawrence Shulman, *Skills of Supervision and Staff Management*. F.E. Peacock Publishers, Itasca, Illinois: 1982, p. 257.

16. The phases of group development identified by William Schwartz are referred to here. See William Schwartz, "Between Client and System: The Mediating Function," pp. 171-197, in Robert W. Roberts and Helen Northen, eds., *Theories of Social Work With Groups*, Columbia University Press, 1976.

17. Wilbert J. McKeachie, *Teaching Tips*, eighth edition, Lexington, Mass.: D.C. Heath and Company, 1986, pp. 53-66.

REFERENCES

Bennis, Warren and Shepard, Herbert. "A Theory of Group Development," *Human Relations*, 1948, Vol. 9, pp. 415-437.

Compton, Beulah and Galaway, Burt. *Social Work Processes*, The Dorsey Press, 1984.

Garland, James, Jones, Hubert and Kolodny, Ralph. "A Model for Stages of Development in Social Work Groups," in Saul Bernstein, ed., *Explorations In Group Work*, 1965.

Gitterman, Alex and Shulman, Lawrence. *Mutual Aid Groups and The Life Cycle*, F.E. Peacock Publishers, 1986.

Goldstein, Howard. *Social Work Practice: A Unitary Approach*, University of South Carolina Press, 1973.

Kadushin, Alfred. *Supervision in Social Work*, Columbia University Press, 1985.

Levinson, Daniel and Klerman, Gerald. "The Clinician-Executive Revisited," *Administration in Mental Health*, 1972, Vol. 6, pp. 53-67.

McKeachie, Wilbert J. *Teaching Tips*, eighth edition, D.C. Heath and Company, 1986.

Northen, Helen. *Social Work With Groups*, Columbia University Press, 1988.

Schwartz, William. "On The Use of Groups in Social Work Practice," in William Schwartz and Serapio Zalba, eds., *The Practice of Group Work*, Columbia University Press, 1971.

Schwartz, William. "Between Client and System: The Mediating Function," in Robert W. Roberts and Helen Northen, eds., *Theories of Social Work With Groups*, Columbia University Press, 1976.

Shulman, Lawrence. *The Skills of Helping Individuals and Groups*, The Peacock Press, 1979.

Shulman, Lawrence. *Skills of Supervision and Staff Management*, F.E. Peacock Publishers, 1982.

Siporin, Max. *Introduction to Social Work Practice*, Macmillan Publishing Company, 1975.

Stempler, Benjamin. "A Group Work Approach To Family Group Treatment," in Albert Alissi, ed., *Perspectives on Social Group Work Practice*, The Free Press, 1980.

Studt, Elliot. "An Outline for Study of Social Authority Factors in Casework," *Social Casework*, 1954, Vol. 35, pp. 231-238.

Studt, Elliot. "Worker-Client Authority Relationships in Social Work," *Social Work*, 1959, Vol. 4, No. 1, pp. 18-28.

Vinter, Robert D. "The Essential Components of Social Group Work Practice," in Robert D. Vinter, ed., *Readings In Group Work Practice*, Campus Publishers, 1967.

Group Empowerment Through Learning Formal Decision Making Processes

John H. Ramey

Empowerment is a major practice approach for work with individuals, families, and communities whether conceived of in clinical, community or other practice frameworks. Analysis of problems leading to the use of empowerment strategies can derive from as divergent theoretical points of view as the worker's selective perception of all or part of the deficit or need of one specific person or group to the radical analysis that all social problems derive from the maldistribution of power. In between, among other analytic frameworks is the developmental analysis that every person and group should learn to use the power necessary to control his/her/their own outcomes or social, economic, and other processes to the maximum degree possible.

Thus, in discussing empowerment, one must be concerned with the ways in which all people, but particularly our client groups participate in the societal decision making processes which determine the distribution of goods and benefits to individuals, groups and communities in our society. The outcome of those decisions is one definition of "social welfare" or social well-being. We know that decisions once made in favor of our client groups will continue to be contested by those from whom the goods and benefits are diverted. Thus they and we have to be prepared to maintain the positions we worked to achieve. It was not by accident that empowerment was a title theme in many of the papers and workshops presented at the 1985 Symposium on Social Work with Groups at Rutgers University and at earlier and later Symposia. It is a very important concept in social work with groups. Our concern in this paper is with groups of adults and teens. Although aspects of formal decision making processes can be used with children's groups, this needs to be discussed in another paper.

Policy decisions are always the outcomes of choices among alternatives. In most sectors they are carried out by various rules ranging from the very informal to the very formal. And the debates are carried out in social units, often small groups such as clubs or committees, but more often larger forums such as township, village, or city councils, children's services boards, state legislatures, or Congress. Even in these latter the basic decision making unit is usually a small task group, such as a committee.

In recent years social work practitioners, researchers, and theorists have emphasized the informal decision making processes. This emphasis was, on the one hand, partly an inherent professional or personal revolt against formalism which avoids personal feelings, partly a lack of education in our schools of social work, and, partly because of the emphasis on the study of interpersonal relationships, the outcomes of interactions in groups and other aspects of group process. There has also been some emphasis in planning and policy practice on alternative formal decision making processes such as Delphi or nominal group processes.

It is our observation that at the higher levels of our society from which the broader policies derive, the decisions are made in a framework of much more formal processes and rules. But many of the current models have not prepared us or our clients for participation in these formal decision making processes.

Further, we as social workers do not usually prepare ourselves or our clients for participation in such processes. As Ephross and Vassil (1988) state, "Many curricula of professional education do not define work group participation as a legitimate part of professional practice." It is our contention that not to do so leaves us and our clients with a power deficit and is in fact a professional disservice. It is proposed here that the group is the social context in which to develop the necessary knowledge and skills for more adequate participation in the formal decision making processes of our political democracy. Group workers need to prepare themselves and their clients not only to participate in but also to provide leadership in such formal processes. The alternative is to rely exclusively on the use of the masses of bodies in protest to influence others to make the correct decisions. In past generations, learning of formal decision making procedures in social agency groups has helped many clients to take constructive leadership roles in society. The social issues leadership vacuum of today is partly an outgrowth of our withdrawal from involvement in leadership training experience in group serving agencies.

As the corporate structure of our society has been rapidly broadening in this century, decisions are increasingly lodged in those fictional, created-in-law persons called corporations. Although created constitutionally or by statute, the Federal and state governments are corporate in structure. Cities are corporations by charter or statute. Counties, townships and villages are corporate chartered subdivisions of the state created by statute. Nongovernmental organizations are corporations, associations, partnerships, or personal and proprietary. Corporations and associations do not exist and therefore can not conduct business except while in session.

In any case, each organization adopts its own rules for conducting business. The Constitution gives each body of Congress the right to adopt its own rules. The same is true for the most part with other levels of government and nongovernment, except that all must conform to constitutional, statutory, regulatory, or case law.

While each organization has sets or rules which may differ, these rules usually have much in common. This is particularly the case since they derive from English Parliamentary procedures developed over the years since the first Parliament was convened in 1258 and the earliest formal treatment of such procedures was written between 1562-66 by Sir Thomas Smyth.

Today the commonly accepted standard for organizations derived from this tradition is *Robert's Rules of Order*. These were first codified by General Henry M. Robert in 1876. He based them on the operating rules of the U.S. House of Representatives, whose rules were then the most common standard. Most organizations have (or should have) in their by-laws an article which reads "Unless otherwise herein provided or required by law, the rules of this organization are those provided in ROBERT'S RULES OF ORDER REVISED and in the latest edition." Absent other applicable rules, if an organizational decision is contested, in general, Robert's Rules will be applied by the courts.

Thus, although various deliberative bodies may have varying rules, Robert's Rules provide a common standard and starting place for learning such procedures. Variations can be dealt with as needed. It should be mentioned here, to be elaborated below, that for smaller organizations or committees, simplified, adapted rules may be used, but they are in the same tradition. And, of course, we should acknowledge the long standing Quaker decision making tradition which requires continuing deliberation until a total consensus is agreed upon. We know of no governmental bodies and only a few nongovernmental organizations which function under these rules.

Henry Robert conceived his Rules of Order in order to achieve certain goals which are, not coincidentally, in direct congruence with social work values. They were designed to insure the survival and enhancement of democracy, to provide for orderly progress from start to finish, to provide for clear focus on the substantive and procedural issues rather than personal issues in organizational meetings, to provide that all minorities and individuals have equal opportunity to participate in the decision making, to provide guidance for the presiding officer fairly to conduct meetings, and to provide for the expeditious completion of the business of the organization. General Robert had found himself as the head of a nongovernmental organization without any coherent codified rules of procedure for carrying out orderly business meetings. So he set forth to create such a body of knowledge. (We will parenthetically note here that, among others, one significant variation of the U.S. Senate Rules is Rule 22 which provides for the filibuster. At that level in government it is probably appropriate ultimately to protect the rights of severely injured minorities, but it is inappropriate at lower levels of organizations.)

In relation to preparation of students and clients for participation in formal decision making processes, we have been asked two questions repeatedly. First, aren't Robert's Rules taught in the schools? Second, is this not an area which belongs in Policy courses or Macro Practice?

In relation to the first, it is our observation that Robert's Rules are taught in the public schools, but that for the most part they are taught at the intellectual level without dealing with the motivations, statuses, or feelings of the persons involved. Further there is little persistence in such instruction with members of minority groups, women, the poor, or other oppressed groups. This failure reinforces the power deficit of these groups and their individual members.

In relation to the second, our response has been that, of course, political decision making is a part of the Policy area, and of Macro Practice. However, we maintain that the basic learning for students should take place in the context of learning how to work with groups, and that, in any case, it is in the group context that learning takes place for the clients. However, if a policy or other macro course is the only place available to provide such instruction, it should be used. It should be noted, however, that such instruction is in the nature of and about group process.

Educating future workers and working with clients in this arena involves similar concerns and processes even though there are significant differences between the classroom and client groups. To be effective both the instructor and the practitioner have to deal with knowledge content, the feelings about the process, and skill development.

Knowledge and skill development will develop through class or group practice. Some important aspects of that will be dealt with below. More important in social work practice is dealing with feelings. Of course, the instructor or worker must have a clear understanding of his or her own feelings and show positive, understanding attitudes toward students and clients. If it is democratic process we are seeking to develop and reinforce, perhaps we should even recognize that the clients own the group and refer to them as members, not clients. This is part of helping persons to feel fully entitled to participate in democratic decision making processes when they may have been socialized to disdain such processes or believe they were not entitled, important or intelligent enough to do so.

Faculty, students and members also have feelings against the formality of the processes. They may have had or been told of experiences in which such processes resulted in persons and groups being injured or otherwise treated inequitably. Or they may have participated in groups where Robert's Rules were handled badly by the chair and the meetings became tangled webs leading to bad decisions. They should be helped to understand that continued failure to learn how to participate and lead such groups will continue to result in injury, injustice, and badly run meetings. Workers need to develop positive attitudes toward formal rules in decision making and to help members to do the same. Most workers and members would not have negative attitudes in relation to the formal rules of football, baseball, basketball or Scrabble. Similarly there are rules in courts where rules are accepted parts of the procedures. A similarly positive attitude has to be developed towards the rules of the decision making processes of deliberative organizations.

There are also feelings about political, economic and other organizational leaders who have used formal rules for their own social, psychological or economic aggrandizement. Of course, there may be a level of self-serving in the use of such rules, but it is most often in the vacuum of inadequate preparation of others to provide a balance of power in such situations.

There are feelings of personal or group inadequacy. "I'm not good enough; I can't learn these rules; my people will never be accepted," etc. Social workers are experts in helping people overcome such attitudes so we will not elaborate techniques here. It is only important to say that systematic, sequential learning of content and skills is necessary, if all else is resolved, to assist in the development of feelings of adequacy and entitlement.

One aspect of this is of importance to instructors and workers. One should not just launch out on one's own into this area of activity. It will be a disservice to members and students if the worker or instructor is not formally educationally prepared for working with Robert's Rules. The knowledge and skill should be there before beginning with a class or group. Courses are available and should be taken to assure thorough preparation.

Several materials are useful for teaching and for working with groups. First, the chart of "All the Rules at a Glance" should be available for all members (Appendix 1). This is a summary of all the motions, the priority ranking of them, and the actions which apply to them. There is a chart which gives the precise wording which should be used to initiate any action (Appendix 2). This is very similar to the signals used in sporting events to indicate an action by the teams, coaches or referees. A statement of abbreviated rules, such as the one published by the League of Women Voters, can also be made available so that it is understood that the full sets of rules do not have to be used in small, more friendly settings. Video training aids are also available. Finally one should have a complete copy of *Robert's Rules of Order, Newly Revised*, for use in reference.

Practice of decision making in the group is the most important feature of learning. Members should have opportunities to play various roles including that of the chairperson, the critical role, in meetings. Particularly, the process of having all conversations take place between members and the chair needs to be learned. This will be difficult for some members and for some social workers who believe that all group processes must allow for free interaction among the members of the group. But it is an important feature of Robert's Rules in their more formal applications in larger assemblies. The informal, interactional processes continue underneath the formal and members must also learn how to use this aspect of the meeting context.

Real group problems may be used for practicing decision making. But it is usually better to use simulations for learning. Thus the dysfunctions in the learning processes do not result in real losses for the group and its members. The simulations can be transformed into games by the creative development of fictional meeting situations in which various decisions are made and in which values are attached to successfully achieving various goals within the meeting.

Limits have to be set regarding the use of the Rules in order to have the game completed. For instance it could not be allowed to move to adjourn right at the beginning in order to defeat the opposition. Such simulations and games are available in the literature of the communications disciplines.

Guests from various decision making units can be brought into a group to explain the importance of learning the Rules and to participate in and to observe various simulations and games. Such guests could be from the United Way, city council, labor union, state legislature, Congress, social agency, association of parliamentarians, Junior Chamber of Commerce, etc. Such persons should be able to give encouragement to members of our groups regarding their adequacy and entitlement to participate in the processes. They should be carefully prepared to help in the learning processes.

Field visits to business meetings of organizations, legislative bodies, unions, etc., should be utilized when such meetings are open or can be made available to observation by groups. Again the preparation is essential. What can be expected? From the outside, without preparation, meetings can appear to be boring, long, tedious, at times. But members can learn, as we have, to observe what is really happening during such intervals in meetings, and to use that knowledge to improve their power in relation to the decisions made in such meetings.

Groups should be encouraged to practice their newly acquired knowledge and skill in the decision making process of their own business meetings. The worker can intervene to assist and make certain that the processes do not become unduly tangled and frustrating. Robert's Rules were designed to enable groups to make decisions efficiently, thoroughly and with full respect for our democratic tradition. We need to be certain that they are used in such a fashion.

Finally, we should act to have members of our groups, with their newly developed skills, appointed and elected to important decision making bodies in our communities. Neighborhood councils are a good place to start. United Way allocations committees are also open to self-nomination for membership. The NAACP and other action groups provide important forums for policy action for persons who have mastered the parliamentary processes.

It must be mentioned in closing that this paper has focused on process. As social workers we must also be aware of the importance of thorough grounding in the content areas of policy and action decisions. Our emphases must be on sound social policies and practices. In a fashion similar to learning the processes, groups can and should learn about important content areas. Such areas may include homelessness, drug use and abuse, abuse of children, spouses, and the elderly, race relations, police protection, community services, and others.

In summary, it is important that we and our clients, the members of groups we work with, learn the rules of formal decision making in order that they can develop the power to participate in the various decision making bodies of our society which determine the distribution of goods and benefits to various individuals and groups, and thus determine their well-being. The small group is an appropriate setting in which to learn and exercise such knowledge and skills. Finally, it is of critical importance that the members of poor, minority, and other oppressed groups and the social workers who serve them learn to participate effectively in such processes so that persons with knowledge and experience of the social problems of our society can bring their concerns more effectively onto the top of our society's agenda once again. Learning the formal rules of decision making is a most important aspect of empowerment.

REFERENCES

Ephross, Paul H., and Thomas V. Vassil. 1988. *Groups That Work: Structure and Process*. New York: Columbia University Press.

Robert, General Henry M. 1984. *Robert's Rules of Order; Newly Revised*. Glenview, Illinois, Scott, Foresman and Company.

APPENDIX I: ALL THE RULES AT A GLANCE

	Motion	Debatable	Amendable	Requires a Second	Vote Required	In Order When Another is Speaking
PRIVILEGED MOTIONS	Time for Next Meeting (when privileged)	No	Yes	Yes	Majority	No
	ADJOURN	No	No	Yes	Majority	No
	Question of Privilege (treat as Main Motion)	Yes	Yes	Yes	Majority	Yes
INCIDENTAL MOTIONS	Point of Order	No	No	No	None unless appealed then Majority	Yes
	Appeal	Yes	No	Yes	Majority	Yes
	Objection to Consideration of Question	No	No	No	2/3	Yes
	Withdrawal of Motion	No	No	No	Majority	No
	Suspension of Rules	No	No	No	2/3	No
	Lay on the Table	No	No	Yes	Majority	No
SUBSIDIARY MOTIONS	Previous Question (close debate)	No	No	Yes	Robert's says 2/3 (majority in many unions)	No
	Limit or Extend Limits of Debate	No	Yes	Yes	Robert's says 2/3 (majority in many unions)	No

Can Be Reconsidered	Motions To Which It Applies	Motions Which Apply To It
No	None	Amend
No	None	None
Yes	None	All
No	Any Motion or Act	None
Yes	Any decision of the chair	Lay on Table, Close Debate, Reconsider
Yes	Main Motion, Any question of privilege	Reconsider
Yes	Any Motion	None
No	Any Motion	None
Yes	Main Motion, Appeals Questions of Privilege, Reconsider	None
Yes	Any Debatable Motion	Reconsider
Yes	Main Motion	Amend, Reconsider, Limit or Close Debate

APPENDIX I: ALL THE RULES AT A GLANCE (Cont'd)

	Motion	Debatable	Amendable	Requires a Second	Vote Required	In Order When Another is Speaking
SUBSIDIARY MOTIONS	Postpone to a Definite Time	Yes	Yes	Yes	Majority	No
	Refer or Commit	Yes	Yes	Yes	Majority	No
	Amend	Yes	Yes	Yes	Majority	No
	Postpone Indefinitely	Yes	No	Yes	Majority	No
	MAIN MOTION	Yes	Yes	Yes	Majority	Yes
	Motion to Reconsider*	Yes, if Motion To Which It Applies Is Debatable	No	Yes	Majority	Yes
	Motion to Rescind*	Yes	Yes	Yes	2/3 or members present; Majority when Notice to rescind was given at previous meeting.	No

*These are treated as if they were main motions.

Can Be Reconsidered	Motions To Which It Applies	Motions Which Apply To It
Yes	Main Motion Question of Privilege	Amend, Reconsider, Limit or Close Debate
Yes	Main Motion Question of	Amend, Reconsider, Limit or Close Debate
Yes	Main Motion Limit Debate Refer, Postpone Fix Time of next meeting	Amend, Reconsider, Close Debate
Yes	Main Motion Question of Privilege	Limit or Close Debate Reconsider
No	None	All
No	Any Motion except adjourn, suspend rules, Lay on Table	Limit Debate, Lay on Table, Postpone Definitely
Yes	Main Motion Appeals, Questions of Privilege	All

APPENDIX 2:
PARLIAMENTARY PROCEDURE...at a glance

TO DO THIS:	YOU SAY THIS:	May you interrupt the speaker?
Adjourn meeting	"I move that we adjourn."	NO
Call an intermission	"I move that we recess for..."	NO
Complain about heat, noise, etc.	"I rise to a question of privilege."	YES
Suspend further consideration of issue	"I move to table the motion."	NO
End debate and amendments	"I move the previous question."	NO
Postpone discussion for a certain time	"I move to postpone the discussion until..."	NO
Give closer study of something	"I move to refer the matter to committee."	NO
Amend a motion	"I move to amend the motion by..."	NO
Introduce business	"I move that..."	NO
THE MOTIONS LISTED ABOVE ARE IN ORDER OF PRECEDENCE... BELOW		
Protest breach of rules or conduct	"I rise to a point of order."	YES
Vote on a ruling of the chair	"I appeal the chair's decision."	YES
Suspend rules temporarily	"I move to suspend the rules so that..."	NO
Avoid considering an improper matter	"I object to the consideration of this motion."	YES
Verify a voice vote by having members stand	"I call for a division," or "Division!"	YES
Request information	"Point of information."	YES
Take up a matter previously tabled	"I move to take from the table..."	NO
Reconsider a hasty motion	"I move to reconsider the vote on"	YES

Notes: (1) Unless a vote is not yet taken.
       (2) Unless the committee has already taken up the subject.
       (3) Only if the motion to be amended is debatable.
       (4) Except in doubtful cases.

Here are some motions you might make,
how to make them and what to expect of the rules.

Do you need a second?	Is it debatable?	Can it be amended?	What vote is needed?	Can it be reconsidered ?
YES	NO	NO	MAJORITY	NO
YES	NO	YES	MAJORITY	NO
NO	NO	NO	NO VOTE	NO (usually)
YES	NO	NO	MAJORITY	NO
YES	NO	NO	2/3	NO (1)
YES	YES	YES	MAJORITY	YES
YES	YES	YES	MAJORITY	YES (2)
YES	YES (3)	YES	MAJORITY	YES
YES	YES	YES	MAJORITY	YES

THERE IS NO ORDER...

NO	NO	NO	NO VOTE (4)	NO
YES	YES	NO	MAJORITY (5)	YES
YES	NO	NO	2/3	NO
NO	NO	NO	2/3 (6)	- (7)
NO	NO	NO	NO VOTE	NO
NO	NO	NO	NO VOTE	NO
YES	NO	NO	MAJORITY	NO
YES	- (8)	NO	MAJORITY	NO

(5) A majority vote in negative to reverse ruling of chair.
(6) A 2/3 vote in negative needed to prevent consideration of main motion.
(7) Only if the main question or motion was not, in fact, considered.
(8) Only if motion to be considered is debatable.

The Social Worker in Politics as a Multi-Role Group Practitioner

Michael Reisch

Despite the historical reluctance of many social workers to dirty their hands in the political process, recently an increasing number are becoming involved in electoral politics as campaign staff and candidates. Their experiences demonstrate the applicability and effectiveness of social work approaches and interventive techniques in an atypical arena. Politics, after all, in the words of former social worker, Senator Barbara Mikulski, is merely "social work with power."

Since electoral campaigns operate largely as a series of loosely knit intergroup activities, the utility of group work methods is of particular relevance to both campaign workers and candidates. In fact, an effective social worker in politics must be able to assume multiple group work roles and apply a broad range of group work concepts. This is because group development, sustenance, coordination and utilization are core tactics of any successful campaign strategy.

DISTINCTIVE FEATURES OF POLITICAL CAMPAIGNS

While social workers in more traditional organizational settings also play multiple group work roles, there are several features of political campaigns which make them distinct in this regard: (1) Social workers are usually not identified as such in the course of campaigns. This generates different expectations of their group role and requires particular sensitivity in the application of group work skills. (2) Political campaigns are of finite duration and have clear outcome objectives which are determined in advance of the initial group work intervention. Nevertheless, there are often periods in which the immediate task environment and the division of roles are characterized by a considerable lack of clarity and ambiguity. The group worker in politics, therefore, must be able to balance the need for focused, task-centered activities with a high degree of short-term uncertainty. (3) The groups with which a worker must be involved in a campaign reflect an unusually wide range of constituent characteristics, a perplexing array of role and status relationships, a varying level of commitment to the project's outcome, and a host of hidden and often conflicting agendas. This places a greater emphasis than usual on the coordination of inter-group activities. (4) The truncated nature of a political campaign, combined with the intensity of the work, and the perpetual climate of scarcity surrounding resources and emotional support, create an atmosphere in which pathological behavior becomes the norm and vice versa. Social work values can often be put to a severe test in such an environment.

Electoral campaigns, therefore, have multiple purposes. Success is defined not only in terms of winning or losing, but also in terms of increasing individual and group participation (through recruitment, involvement and empowerment of community members); enhancing public awareness of issues (education); creating new resources for present and future utilization (volunteers, money, contributors, mailing lists, and skilled staff); and developing and strengthening political organizations and groups.

In addition, political campaigns involve an innovative process of group development in which organizations are built around familiar institutions such as neighborhoods, community or civic associations, and labor unions. Utilizing the familiar as a bridge to participation in a new organizational entity (the campaign), enhances a campaign's capacity to identify and build upon natural or pre-existing loyalties; gather information; identify and recruit those groups to whom outreach efforts are likely to be receptive; locate and develop group leaders; neutralize potential "hostiles"; build communication networks with new groups; and learn group customs, values and symbols more quickly in order to incorporate them into the campaign.

Finally, the groups which are created within a political campaign are different in several ways from those with which social workers are accustomed. They are time limited, rather than open-ended. They are often focused on the needs of a primary individual–the candidate–who is outside the group. They require different roles of the staff responsible for organizing, leading and facilitating them.

TYPES OF GROUPS IN POLITICAL CAMPAIGNS

The range of groups in a political campaign is enormous, reflecting the diverse tasks which must be undertaken to create a successful effort. Groups include pre-existing groups, both natural and formed, and groups which are created specifically for the campaign and which cease to exist upon its conclusion.

Pre-existing groups include political clubs and party organizations, unions and professional associations, churches, political action committees, business organizations, consultant firms, "good government" groups, and other campaign organizations. Obviously, because each of these groups is needed for a different purpose in the campaign's development, different approaches are required when working with them individually or in combinations.

Groups that are specifically created for political campaigns are also quite varied. They tend to fall into two categories, formal and informal. Most campaign organizations utilize a formal structure consisting of three group levels.

The Operating or Executive Committee

This group meets regularly to develop overall campaign strategy. It includes people from both inside and outside the campaign and is led by the campaign manager or a preselected chairperson. In some circumstances, the candidate will be the official or unofficial leader of this group. In general, this is not advisable as s/he often lacks the time and the perspective to make the hard decisions which this group must make.

The Advisory Committee

This group, which meets about once every two months, functions as a broad sounding board for campaign strategy and themes. Ideally, it is comprised of at least one representative from each constituent group with which the campaign is involved. The titular group leader should be selected from a "second line" or emerging group. The goals of this group are leadership development and serving as a conduit for community feedback about the campaign and its various components, such as ads, literature, themes, and issues. Unlike the Executive Committee, with which the candidate meets regularly, the candidate is present only at the initial meeting of the Advisory Committee and at annual symbolic meetings thereafter.

The Coordinating Committee

Unlike the Advisory Committee in which the emphasis is on process, this group is highly task-oriented. It requires the ongoing involvement of a consistent core of people who represent the various elements of the campaign. To ensure optimal functioning, the participants in this group should be the highest level official from each part of the campaign (e.g., fundraising, field operations, publicity). The purpose of the Advisory Committee is to avoid duplication of effort, role conflicts and turf battles which might arise, and to apply campaign resources efficiently particularly in regard to voter registration, get-out-the-vote, literature distribution, and public appearances.

Two major informal groups develop in every political campaign. One consists of the office staff in the campaign headquarters. Because this staff is comprised of both paid and volunteer workers, there are some potential tensions about roles, work distribution and status that need to be addressed regularly. The other informal group is the campaign's "inner circle," which includes the candidate and key campaign advisors. This group is often quite small and is usually characterized by the longevity of the participants' relationships. Problems for the campaign may emerge when a newcomer, for example a campaign manager, "joins" this group as a matter of necessity, or when the decisions of this group come into conflict with those of the campaign's Executive Committee.

Campaign groups, as social groups, experience many of the same traits as their counterparts in the more familiar surroundings of social service agencies. They reflect the social status of the community, while creating their own status and role hierarchy in the decision making process. They experience conflict and demonstrate the need to exercise control both internally and over their external environment. They contain both an interpersonal structure and a task or division of labor structure. These groups create their own decision making process and style. They also develop and sustain their own traditions, and a distinctive group morale or esprit. The social climate of these groups varies, generally falling somewhere on the continuum between authoritarian and democratic. They are never laissez-faire.

THE ROLE OF THE WORKER

The role of the social worker with these groups—as campaign manager or field operations director, in particular—is similar to that played in social service settings. S/he is alternately an organizer, mediator, leader, facilitator, mobilizer, coordinator, and problem solver. The confusing part for the worker is that these different roles must often be performed in the same day with little time for reflection or self-evaluation. A particularly difficult situation arises when the worker must meet with two or more groups simultaneously, with which s/he has played very different roles. Three issues are particularly adaptable from social group work to political work: autonomy, mediation, and group resistance.

The autonomy of each group within a campaign varies to a considerable extent, depending upon the level of skill of its members, their prior experience in politics, the degree of interpersonal trust which exists between the group members, and the group's allegiance to the campaign. To maximize the campaign's chances for success, certain group goals and behaviors must be prescribed. Within these parameters, however, the worker should give each group latitude to express differences in style and tactics. This enables the group to "own" the process and develop a sense of itself as a decision making body. It also contributes to the group's internal cohesion and effectiveness and its connectedness to the overall campaign. Lastly, it is more likely to create a climate in which the group members feel empowered by their participation.

Group resistance is a knotty problem for the political group worker. Resistance is particularly likely from preestablished groups over turf issues, campaign style, and control of resources. It may also occur in new groups based on members' uncertainty, fear of risk, personal stress, and fear of loss of individual or group identity in the course of the campaign.

There are a number of tactics a worker can utilize to help overcome this resistance. First, the worker can strive to motivate group members based on their perception of need rather than goals dictated by an external body. To do this, the group must be involved in the decision making process from its inception. Where necessary, use peer pressure of sympathetic group members to create group cohesion and promote cooperation. Second, the worker needs to be sensitive to the pressures each group member experiences as a result of his/her participation in the campaign pressures of time, of risk, and of involvement in new and somewhat initially mysterious activities. The worker should address the potentially adverse consequences of participation on family life, physical and emotional well-being, and social relationships at the outset. Shortly after the group has been formed, s/he should also discuss the long-term (post-campaign) effects of participation on the group and its members.

The worker should establish reasonable objectives for the group based upon a thorough assessment of the group's capabilities. Once these objectives have been determined, the worker should allow for some flexibility in adjusting them as the realities of the campaign temper the enthusiastic aspirations of group participants. These realities also require, however, that commitments must be honored and that group members will be held accountable for what they do and do not do. The worker, therefore, should expect open, explicit commitments from the group and utilize the group itself to hold group members to their various commitments.

Above all, the worker should remember that respect and appreciation for group members are critical aspects of the campaign process. Respect requires that the worker emphasize cohesive values, behave in a consistent manner, and never equivocate in his/her actions. Appreciation is demonstrated through the use of symbolic rewards and by holding interim celebrations throughout the campaign.

Unlike social group work, however, the campaign worker's goals are determined by the requirements of the campaign itself and the candidate's wishes, rather than that of the various group participants. When conflicts arise, it is important to resolve them internally, therefore, at the lowest possible organizational level, involving as few people as possible. The worker's legitimacy and power varies with each group with whom s/he works. It is most legitimate and most powerful with those groups the worker has helped form and with those intergroup "coalitions" the worker has initiated. Ironically, these are also two of the most difficult tasks for the worker to perform. In each of the worker's tasks, the key element is the transfer of the worker's, legitimacy, power, and skills to the group and its members (as well as the resources the group needs to complete its tasks) within the focus of the overall goals of the campaign.

GROUP DEVELOPMENT IN POLITICAL CAMPAIGNS

The process of group and intergroup development in political campaigns is both similar to and different from the experience of groups with which most social workers are accustomed. The differences are, in general, consequences of the political process itself which affect such essential group characteristics as time, membership composition, available resources, group objectives, and relationship to the group worker/facilitator.

Five significant differences can, therefore, be identified: (1) The stages of group development in political campaigns are often because of the campaign's schedule. (2) Different groups within a campaign have different "timeliness" for their particular tasks, have been in existence for different lengths of time, and have "life expectancies" which range from permanent to very short-term. (3) Different groups within a campaign, therefore not only have different purposes and functions, but also different styles and composition. (4) With regard to the purposes for involvement in the campaign itself, some groups see the candidate's election as their sole or primary raison d'être. Others regard the election as part of a broader issue-oriented or organization-building strategy. Still others see the campaign as an unavoidable distraction from more important activities. Such varying motivations complicate the group role of the worker. (5) Political campaigns need to plan their activities by "thinking backwards," from election day to the initial period of group formation. This changes the way in which groups establish goals and the manner in which group resources are budgeted. It is also important to note that the phases of group development in a campaign are not as clearly distinct as in most social groups and, of particular importance to the worker, that different campaign groups are at different stages of development at the same time.

STAGES OF DEVELOPMENT IN CAMPAIGN GROUPS

Aside from these above-mentioned differences, the stages of group development in a political campaign–pre-planning, formation, maturity/coordination, and termination–closely resemble those of other social groups. In the discussion below, the focus will be on those groups which are created specifically for the campaign, including those which are formed by merging pre-existing groups. The discussion omits the role of the worker with pre-existing groups whose internal structure is scarcely affected by participation in the campaign.

The Pre-Planning Stage

In this stage the worker must assess the political "baggage" of group participants, their social context, political experience, relationship to the candidate and the campaign's issues, the group's current strength and interests, and its level of tension and anxiety in comparison with other political experiences in its past.

As with treatment groups, the worker must identify the benefits and risks of individual and group involvement (short-term and long-term) for both the group and the campaign. In addition, it is important to identify the specific goals and objectives for the group's participation in the campaign.

The worker should recognize that individuals and groups will vary in the aspects of political involvement that they find most attractive. For some, the opportunity to express their views before a wider audience is critical; for others, the attraction may lie in the sense of belonging to an entity larger than themselves. The key task is to develop incentives and alternative means to attract and retain group participation. This not only legitimates the different motives, values and emphases of different groups, it is more democratic and empowering.

The worker needs to be aware that although the "tone" of any campaign group, its leadership and decision making style, reflect its unique composition, purpose, and dynamics, it must also be sensitive to the needs of the campaign at all times. Despite the pressure this realization creates, above all the worker must be patient, recognizing that different groups move at different paces. While patience is often difficult to put into practice during a stressful political campaign, it is vital if the worker is to learn from both successes and failures.

Group Origins

Just as with treatment groups in a clinical setting, if the worker is utilizing "natural" groups s/he needs to be clear about the group's background and purposes. In the case of new groups, it is particularly important to specify the group's purposes as clearly as possible from the outset.

People get involved in campaigns in much the same way as they get involved in therapy groups: they are referred by another individual or organization; they are self-referred in response to an ad, a piece of organizational literature, or something they saw in the media; or they join a campaign group because of the recruitment efforts of the worker. Similarly, individuals participate in a campaign for varied and multiple reasons, such as personal or group gain or recognition, as a means of solving, deflecting, or escaping from problems or pressures.

Some of the factors which affect the motivation of an individual to participate in a political group include: his/her values, which are shaped by personal and community status and provide the individual with a political frame of reference; the individual's environment, especially family and work; other reference groups in the individual's life; personal capabilities; previous experience with politics; and the individual's prior impressions of the candidate, the campaign, the worker or politics itself, which may be obtained either through personal experience or the community "grapevine." All of these factors constitute the "baggage" which individuals and groups bring to the campaign.

The specific reasons that an individual or group becomes involved in a political campaign at a particular "point of entry," however, may be irrelevant to the campaign's objectives. The critical task for the worker, therefore, is to convert these motives into actions which simultaneously contribute positively to the campaign and satisfy (or, at the very least, do not alienate) the group participants. With regard to satisfaction, natural or pre-existing groups may be more easily integrated into the campaign than newly formed groups. Such groups, however, may also be less able to adjust their goals and behaviors to the needs of the campaign. For the worker, they represent a necessary but problematic resource.

The Formative Stage

This is the stage of a campaign where interpersonal ties are created and lasting links to a campaign are forged. In this stage, leadership roles in campaign groups are established, and commonalities with new and old groups are identified. It is, therefore, a crucial stage for the success of a political campaign. Using familiar group work language, this stage can be divided into exploratory and bargaining phases.

The key in the exploratory phase is the exchange of information and the development of group goals specific to the campaign. The campaign worker must be careful not to dominate the newly formed group (or the group whose allegiance to the campaign is new) and remember to be patient with all groups. The worker must recognize group members' past and potential contributions and skills, and their connections to other potential group members, supporters and contributors. (It is important to note here that unlike some social work groups in service settings, a campaign group is always looking for new members.)

It is also important to be clear in this phase about campaign goals and the roles of individuals and groups in attaining them. This means that the worker should leave no room for ambiguity in identifying group objectives and group tasks. To facilitate this result, the worker should encourage the group to develop a formal list of priorities (where multiple goals exist) and to develop a schedule for attaining them, keeping in mind that a campaign always thinks "backwards" from Election Day. One tool that is helpful in developing such a schedule is a human resources budget that keeps in mind both the ebb and flow of campaign activities and the need to "pace" individuals who work within it.

Sometimes a worker's connection with a group will be solely through its leaders. This is particularly true in the case of natural or pre-existing groups. Such groups are also more likely to determine their own pattern of task allocation once the overall tasks for the group within the campaign are identified.

The bargaining phase in a campaign is especially important with pre-existing groups. In fact, in many campaigns it is often an ongoing feature of inter-group relations. This bargaining will occur over resources, rewards, status, power, and the scheduling of activities. Negotiation with established groups is particularly difficult if one is a newcomer to campaigns. A new campaign director or campaign functionary often feels that s/he "lost" in the negotiation process in early bargaining sessions, whatever the outcome. Under such circumstance it is best to adopt the role of a learner without revealing one's ignorance of the intricacies of the political bargaining process. Sometimes it is helpful to consult with veteran allies prior to a difficult bargaining session. They may be able to clarify potential outcomes of the session, and thereby provide guideposts as to what can reasonably be expected from the negotiations.

In new groups the development of priorities must be done with a specific focus on the campaign, while taking into account the group members' needs and abilities. The key is to strive to maximize the participation of both individuals within the group and the group within the campaign.

Disagreements in this phase are inevitable, especially with pre-existing groups. It is best to identify, confront and try to resolve such disagreements early in the campaign as tensions will invariably mount later, and the time to resolve them gets much shorter. The key is to remember that since unanimity is not necessary for success, the worker should identify those issues around which agreement is essential and those around which "cooperative disagreement," concessions, or compromise are acceptable. For example, there should be no disagreement about a campaign's message; but how that message is communicated to a particular group of voters can be open to discussion and different interpretation.

In both types of groups the task orientation of a campaign requires the creation of a clear group structure. It is important, however, to avoid isolating the parts from the whole at all levels of a campaign. One way to avoid this is through sub-group presentations at meetings. Another is to build in group liaisons with a campaign steering or coordinating committee.

The Coordination Stage

This stage can last anywhere from several months to nearly a year in political campaigns. Usually a campaign rhythm develops as group norms and processes are established and implemented and group tasks are allocated. Ideally, the group should "peak" as a cohesive and productive entity in the last phase of a campaign the final several weeks before the election. One potential obstacle to the development of this cohesion is the emergence of factions within or between campaign groups.

Factionalism

Within each campaign group there are opposing elements that can strengthen or weaken its potential growth and contribution to the campaign. A cohesive group can become fragmented if tasks are not clearly established. Conversely, a demoralized group can be energized by a successful activity at a critical moment in the campaign.

A campaign worker can take several steps to reduce the development of factionalism with campaign groups. Building trust among the members of the group and between the group and the campaign as a whole is primary. This means that a worker should never lie to the group, although it is sometimes necessary for tactical purposes to withhold information. Secondly, the campaign worker must be alert to the sources and composition of potential factions and actively intervene at group meetings to discourage their development. The latter can be accomplished in several ways:

- by focusing meetings on information sharing, skill development and organizational growth;
- by encouraging selection of a chair who is able to remain impartial and is not identified with any particular existing or emerging faction;
- by establishing from the outset that group decisions will be made by consensus, rather than voting;
- by utilizing a clear, future and action-oriented agenda;
- by delegating both authority and responsibility as widely as possible within the group;
- by creating an environment full of socialization, pleasantness and, above all, fun (especially in the latter stages of a campaign when everyone is tired and pressured);
- by adjusting the aspirations of the group and members if initial goals are unrealistic (either too high or too low) or a gap emerges between the aspirations of the group and certain individuals within it.

Goal Implementation and Evaluation

In a political campaign, in which group behavior is adjusting constantly to changing circumstances, goal implementation and evaluation are ongoing and complementary processes. In the course of a campaign, particularly one that is hotly contested, evaluation becomes more critical even as it becomes more difficult. Knowing this, a successful campaign should try to build in evaluative processes wherever feasible. One way to do this is by "checking in" with the campaign group regularly, on both a formal and informal basis. Another is to schedule periodic meetings for purposes of obtaining feedback and boosting campaign morale. A third technique, if resources allow, is to distribute a regular campaign newsletter.

It is important to note that many group members are involved elsewhere even during the most active stages of a campaign. Realization of the multiple roles and responsibilities of group members requires a campaign worker to separate the evaluation of the task performance of the group(s) over which s/he has responsibility from the effects the campaign is having on the group's members, while simultaneously understanding how the environment in which group members live and work influences the group's assessment of its goal attainment which, in turn, affects its ability to reach its goals.

The Termination Stage

All campaigns, however successful, must come to an end. That is both a bane and a blessing of political work. In creating campaign groups, it is important to be clear from the outset about whether the group is expected to end when the campaign is over, or whether it is expected to continue to function in some fashion between campaigns (for example, to serve as a conduit for issue generation, an instrument for volunteer recruitment for subsequent campaigns, or a means to raise campaign funds). The reality of late 20th century American politics is that some campaign groups must be perpetually maintained to keep the structure and the spirit of the campaign alive, and to ensure the future prospects of the candidate.

CONCLUSION

More than at any time in this century, politics and the human services are inextricably connected. Social workers and the programs and policies for which they stand are confronted by serious challenges at the national, state and local levels. Politics is no longer an activity which social workers can escape by hiding behind a veil of professionalism. This essay has attempted to demystify the politics of an electoral campaign by demonstrating that social work skills in group development and group process can be readily transferred to another arena. If the psychological obstacles to political participation can be overcome, social workers will then possess both the tools and the mindset needed for successful political intervention. In acquiring these new tools and this different view of themselves and the world of politics, it is also likely they will become better practitioners in the more familiar surroundings of social service agencies.

The Telephone Group:
Accessing Group Service
to the Homebound

Lynne Stein
Beulah Rothman
Manuel Nakanishi

Relatively little is known about the use of telephone groups for populations who normally cannot avail themselves of groupwork services. Such populations primarily consist of persons who are homebound because of illness or disability or are geographically removed from others like themselves. Their need for social supports and/or therapeutic groupwork experience are largely unmet. The telephone group is an innovative response to filling this gap.

While only a few articles on telephone groups have been published these have reported on the effectiveness of telephone groups with the elderly blind (Evans and Jaureguy, 1981; Evans and Jaureguy, 1982; Evans, Werkhoven, Fox and Halar, 1982; Jaureguy and Evans, 1983); chronically disabled (Evans, 1986; Evans, Fox, Pritzl and Halar, 1984; Evans, Kleinman, Halar and Herzen, 1984); and handicapped college students (Kennard and Shilman, 1979; Shilman and Giladi, 1985).

Reduction of isolation, support for coping with present and future losses in functioning, freedom from total dependence on others within the immediate environment, and understanding and empathy from fellow sufferers are some of the therapeutic gains attributed to telephone groups.

In general, the telephone group is characterized as a conference call with five to seven participants including the worker. It is a closed group communicating on a regular basis and is facilitated within the framework of social groupwork.

203

This paper consolidates existing practice knowledge and findings gleaned from written literary accounts, a simulated telephone group created for the purpose of orienting the authors to the service, and an actual telephone group of persons with multiple sclerosis facilitated by a professional social group worker.

INITIAL CONCERNS

Technical and mechanical concerns loom as major issues for the groupwork practitioner inexperienced with the workings of a telephone group. How costly is the service? Can it operate within any telephone system? Is special equipment necessary and where can technical consultation be obtained? In addition, professional questions arise from unfamiliarity with the telephone as a therapeutic medium and from distrust of it as an amplifier of meaningful interpersonal communication. Irritation with the depersonalization of the ubiquitous telephone answering message machine and the intrusive hard-sell promotional call have conditioned our views of the telephone as a non-nurturing instrument. Is it risky to start a telephone group for vulnerable clients who have no other social supports? Will these clients be further isolated and dehumanized by the lack of visual contact and detachment of the telephone vacuum? Is special knowledge and competence required to work with such a group? How perceptive and responsive can the practitioner be to an anonymous, faceless, group of individuals? Professional uneasiness is evoked by such questions, but they need not deter the group worker from creating the telephone group, an essential service for those without an opportunity for a group experience.

THE SIMULATED TELEPHONE GROUP SESSION

The utility of simulation as a means of anticipating new experiences and challenges has been long appreciated by social group workers. Unsure of the road ahead, and interested in forming a telephone group as an agency service for multiple sclerosis persons, the leading author of this paper enlisted the aid of a neighboring school of social work to simulate a telephone group session. The two faculty authors of this paper and three students participated in a simulated telephone session in order to better understand the dynamics of a therapeutic telephone group. The simulation team assumed the roles of multiple sclerosis persons characterized as middle-aged and chronically afflicted by the illness for more than ten years. All but one had spouses who had abandoned them, all were wheelchair-bound, confined to their homes, too frail to attend a community-based group, and most had infrequent interpersonal contacts. These roles and circumstances are not atypical for chronically ill homebound multiple sclerosis persons.

In preparation for the first meeting of the simulated telephone group, the team met in advance to review their concerns and expectations in order to heighten their awareness of the elements of the pending process. The team was cognizant of their dual role as participant and observer. They needed to systematically note the process and the dynamics they would be experiencing, and to transmit this information to the practitioner.

Importantly, the simulated group session took place under conditions closely approximating the "real thing." Simulation team members participated in the group sessions from the privacy of their own homes or office. The group worker placed the call through the conference operator, and checked on the auditory conditions for each member and the group as a whole.

As a result of the orientation, the simulation team had no difficulty in assuming role identities and in suggesting working principles to the practitioner which could be useful in the forthcoming real telephone group. For the inexperienced practitioner contemplating development of telephone group service, a simulation is an excellent orienting exercise and is recommended. The experience offered direct assurance that a telephone group could be rewarding for the group members and the practitioner. The enthusiasm of the team may have resulted from the "halo effect," but the simulation energized the practitioner and increased her motivation not only to facilitate a single telephone group, but also to develop a telephone service program on an agency-wide basis. The simulation was a small investment given the benefits derived from it.

BEGINNING THE GROUP: MECHANICS

The first task confronting the practitioner is locating the appropriate service from the telephone company. This can be obtained by contacting the business office in the specific locale and requesting a conference call operator. The operator is given a list of the participant's telephone numbers (not to exceed the conference call limitation of the local area), as well as the exact time the call will be placed to each party. Call arrangements must be predetermined with participating group members prior to the call. At the time of the call, each member is contacted and awaits the phone call until all parties are connected. Geographic distance of participants does not impact on the strength of communication. The telephone company must be informed as to the originating party for billing purposes. In this instance, the agency assumed financial responsibility for providing this service, however, alternate billing procedures can be used according to the needs of the group and the provider. Charges for a one hour call are extremely reasonable if all participants reside in the same county. For example, as a guide to the practitioner, the AT&T system charges were between ten and twelve dollars for a one hour call for five persons within the same county. Rates may differ in other areas.

If the participant has a call waiting feature on his/her phone, it must be ignored during the telephone session. Individual amplifiers should also be avoided because they tend to distort voices and are annoying to the group. As an alternative, for those who cannot hold the telephone for a lengthy period of time an inexpensive shoulder apparatus can be purchased. If needed, technical consultation is available through the local telephone company.

SELECTION OF MEMBERS

Group members were recruited from a newsletter mailed to all registered members of the agency. Intake interviews were then conducted by telephone by the practitioner to screen members for homogeneity with regard to their handicap. Information was obtained about the member's endurance, particularly the ability to hold the telephone for a period of one hour. In assessing persons with multiple sclerosis, overall strength is a critical dimension. The physical capabilities of homebound members who would participate in a telephone group should be carefully evaluated. Most home-bound persons, regardless of the etiology of their handicap, will probably have some physical limitation or deterioration which can affect participation.

Verbal and cognitive skills were also evaluated. One basic condition of the contract was the expectation that members would participate verbally. Verbal facility was determined as necessary by the practitioner, particularly in view of the fact that this was the first telephone group in the agency. However, in a telephone group of homebound college students, verbal facility for all members was not necessary. The group worker acted as moderator and interpreter for two members who had serious speech impediments (Shilman and Giladi, 1985).

During this initial intake interview, there were several other conditions that were agreed upon; the members were requested to sign a release from liability on the part of the agency, members were expected to make a six week commitment to participate in the group, and all calls made outside of the telephone group, amongst the members at other times, were to be paid by them.

The purpose of the group, in the intake interview, was interpreted broadly to be a closed mutual support group with insured confidentiality. The concepts of networking and mutual aid were discussed. Most importantly, opportunities for communicating with others and breaking through the silence of their lives were the primary foci of presenting and accepting the telephone group. Thus, the major objectives were to reduce loneliness and stress to promote a more positive outlook.

Specifically, during the intake interview the practitioner determined with each member a convenient schedule for the group call and enough information about each person to "tune in" to the needs of the members and their potential participation within the group.

The following briefly describes the members selected for the first telephone group. Dr. S. resides in a skilled nursing facility. He was the youngest resident in the home and there were no other persons to whom he can relate. He is totally dependent on staff for his care.

Scheduling with the cooperation of the nursing home was essential to guarantee that he would be in his bed to receive the call. Dr. S.'s hobby is writing poetry.

Mr. B. was completely confined to his home. Aside from the multiple sclerosis, the most significant event in his life is his wife's abandonment after a marriage of thirty-eight years. Mr. B.'s anger with his wife is pervasive. He feels he has been given a "bum rap."

Mrs. C. had been bed-bound for several years. She lives with her son and is totally dependent on him for her daily living activities. This is an unsatisfactory arrangement as the reversal of roles creates stress and anger.

Mrs. M. was the youngest member in the telephone group. She is recently divorced after twenty-two years of marriage and has moved back with her mother. Compared to the other members of the group, her home situation offers considerable support.

The fifth member, Miss E., despite encouragement and support by the practitioner, dropped out of the group prior to the first session. She claimed she was unable to make a six week commitment, although she initially agreed to join.

The group's members were similar with regard to their predicament. The unifying characteristic sustaining the group was the handicap of the members and their need for social intercourse. The heterogeneity of other attributes; gender, ethnicity, religion and education, were relatively insignificant.

GROUP PROCESS

Initially participants needed help in identifying themselves and others by voice. The practitioner reinforced connections between names and voices. The necessity of this assistance, however, was surprisingly short-lived. Members and practitioner were quick to make the accurate associations between person and voice.

Telephone group participants exhibited many of the customary beginning patterns of interaction found in face-to-face groups. Ambivalence has to be resolved, commonalities established, the authority conflict worked through, normative expectations and structures introduced, and trust developed. The issue of confidentiality emerged again and moved to the forefront in the first session. When and where members and worker were located during the telephone session was of paramount importance. Each member and the worker was required by the group to be in a secluded environment during the telephone session. The demand for privacy appeared to be a critical dimension in balancing member control with worker authority. Discussion of privacy and confidentiality provided the foundation for auditory intimacy and trust.

Different conceptions of how members perceived and articulated the purposes of the group were gently explored in the first session. Anticipating that the commonality of despair could be overwhelming, the practitioner focused on the excitement of the new experience–the group. She supported the members' sense of uniqueness from other multiple sclerosis persons who did not have the benefit of membership in a telephone group. The novelty of using something so commonplace as the telephone to open up a world that had been closed to them appealed to the imagination of the members. Homebound persons depressed with their life situation are able to appreciate and enjoy new challenges. The telephone group offers an adventure in communication.

The telephone group can take many forms with regard to structure and process. In this particular group an unstructured format was viewed by the practitioner as being the most desirable. The practitioner assessed that flexibility seemed appropriate. A highly structured group for people denied normal social intercourse imposes constraints which are premature and limiting. An emerging process mode of group format, as identified in the Mainstream Model of group work (Papell and Rothman, 1979), seemed preferable with persons with diminished empowerment. Thus, themes discussed in every telephone session essentially flowed from individual members' perceived interests and needs, and were synthesized as group themes in the interventions employed by the worker. In this regard, reframing a problem and reaching for members' interests were the principal interventions utilized by the practitioner.

Efforts to contain dysfunctional hopelessness in the group did not preclude recurrent themes of dependency, depression, loneliness and inactivity as themes for group discussion. However, focus on mutual aid and bringing to their awareness the members' capacities

to assist each other with problem solving helped to prevent a debili-
tating contagion of depression in the group. Reframing the problem
while most frequently utilized, other interventions such as external-
izing the problem, universalizing, labeling feelings and prioritizing
alternatives, were also employed by the worker.

Group members were encouraged to provide assistance to each
other to tackle simple activities of daily living routines to promote
more independence. The realization that regaining some control
over one's life and decreasing dependency even in small measures,
contributed to heightening self-confidence of the members. Sharing
of information and feedback from group members became expect-
able activity in processing any problem introduced in the group.

Mr. B. was helped by the group in two critical incidents. He had
fallen in the shower and was helpless for several hours. The trauma
was shared by the group. While sympathetic, the group chose alternative ways in the future to avoid a recurrence of this incidence. At
another session Mr. B. needed help in resolving a conflict with his
daughter. In both instances Mr. B. felt the support of the group and
expressed appreciation. Recognition of the group's ability to help
Mr. B. was the turning point for the group. It fostered more intense
feelings of intimacy and sharing, and created an atmosphere of
trust.

During the course of the group, members revealed an extensive
knowledge about their illness. Discussions related to multiple sclerosis dealt with the uncertainty of disease progression, anxiety over
recurrent exacerbations, treatment modalities, frustration with unsuccessful research and lack of a cure. A pervasive fantasy which
was not dispelled by knowledge or group discussion was the belief
that in some way the multiple sclerosis persons caused the illness,
or there was something the person might have done to prevent it.
Any attempt by the practitioner to correct this perception was not
accepted by individual members. It was essentially shrugged off by
them.

Two group activities were experimentally introduced by the practitioner to determine the use of program in a telephone group. The
first was designed to focus on mental ability rather than physical
disability. The members were encouraged to compose an original
piece of work which would describe feelings about the telephone

group. Two members produced a poem and a song. While the activity was task-oriented, the purpose was to emphasize that reduction in physical mobility was not necessarily congruent with loss of cognitive ability. The group experienced a sense of pride and identity with the accomplishment and creative ability of the two members.

The second activity was an exchange of photographs amongst the group members and the practitioner. The members resisted this exchange at first but were encouraged by the worker to contribute their photo. The pictures confirmed the physical disabilities of the members and introduced the visual reality of their illness. The initial resistance of the members to the exchange of photographs was not correctly assessed by the worker. The impact of this activity called attention to the possibility that chronically handicapped persons may be sensitive to the diminution of physical attractiveness. The members may have been hesitant to reveal real or assumed deterioration to others. In retrospect, this activity may have been premature and prompted more by the need of the practitioner to establish a stronger and more comfortable reality base for the group and herself.

The use of program can be utilized as a source of enrichment to help break through isolation, and also, serve a therapeutic value to further develop the individual's self-esteem. The group's appreciation of Dr. S.'s poetry was a powerful validation of his ability to overcome his predicament. However, in considering program activity, group development and the subjective meaning of the activity to the members, needs should be carefully appraised. For example, reality testing as functional for most groups may be assessed somewhat differently where the development of fantasy is a more appropriate defense. The question for the practitioner in the telephone group remains: Is it of merit to focus on reality or keep the illusions of fantasy present?

ROLE OF THE WORKER

At the outset, the affective quality of the practitioner's voice creates the climate of the telephone group. The practitioner relies solely on his/her ability to communicate by voice alone, to stimulate participation, encourage interaction, convey recognition and acceptance of individual members, and to project a vision of the group as a whole. There is an intensity of concentration on the part of the practitioner on the auditory stimuli. Without visual cues, demands are placed on the worker to be highly sensitive to participants' affect and to sustain the flow of conversation to include all members. Long lapses of conversation by one member creates discomfort for the others. It is as if the silent member is eavesdropping on the others. The practitioner is called upon to be an intermediary to either move in on the silence or to indirectly involve the nonparticipant. In such situations the practitioner needs to rely on intuition to respond to the unspoken messages that are not being communicated.

Unlike the face-to-face group, simultaneous discussions are intolerable in the telephone group. The worker must intervene quickly to head off chaos and confusion. However, a strong similarity does exist with the face-to-face group when a single member monopolizes the meeting time and the attention of the group. This is particularly critical since the worker cannot assess the reactions of other members when one member is holding center stage for too long a period of time. Delayed intervention can be a disadvantage in these circumstances.

SPECIAL ASPECTS

One negative aspect of the telephone group is client and practitioner fatigue. Holding the telephone receiver for a long period of time can be exhausting. Relying on a single sense for communication can produce overload. The practitioner must check the fatigue level periodically throughout the session and can be guided by the members' suggestions on optimal length of meeting time. The practitioner is also not immune from this effect and needs to be aware of possible fatigue on her part as well.

The telephone group requires disciplined use of time by the practitioner. There is no margin of time for the proverbial "doorknob" discussion familiar in the face-to-face group. Time limitations are predetermined and the practitioner needs to prepare herself and the group for appropriately ending each session.

The absence of face-to-face contact is conducive to the development of fantasies, as discussed previously, by the group members and the practitioner. As a consequence, feelings of dissociation from reality, loss of control in the group situation and other such irrational responses may occur from time to time by the practitioner or the group members. Such reactions can be anticipated and need not stimulate excessive anxiety.

TERMINATION

It is helpful at the outset if the practitioner is clear about termination, the limits of agency service, possible renegotiation of the length of the telephone group contract, potential for transformation to a self-help group and the nature of agency responsibility should the group continue independently. The multiple sclerosis group was terminated after six weeks which conformed to the original agreement with the members. Unfortunately, due to limitations of agency budget, the group was unable to continue. There was concern on the part of the practitioner that six weeks was too short a time period to achieve a more substantial degree of bonding that could provide for longer term affiliation and support. If additional resources had been available, a more optimal period of ten weeks would have been recommended. This would allow for exploring in greater depth the members' continuing their association. In this group the members' desire to continue their contact was relatively unattended. The practitioner did provide a list of telephone numbers to all of the members and encouraged continuation of the natural and positive relationships that had developed during the course of the group, but she was unable to play a facilitating role in helping the members implement a plan in this regard.

CONCLUSION

Experience with the multiple sclerosis telephone group provided many answers to the questions raised at the beginning of this paper that were in the minds of the simulation team and the practitioner. This group documented that homebound persons greatly benefit from telephone group contact and professional group service. Group members are able to rapidly accommodate to the telephone instrument and compensate for lack of visual contact. They are able to communicate affectively and develop emotional support. The practitioner, although experiencing some discomfort with the anonymity of the members, also rapidly accommodates to limited cues. The sensitivity and the skills normally brought by the practitioner into any group program were readily available and effective in the multiple sclerosis telephone group.

Telephone group service has tremendous potential for the social work profession to reach out to many different populations and persons who are homebound. It provides an inexpensive means of networking individuals who have no other opportunity to participate in other groupwork services and activities. As practitioners continue to use this medium, increased competence and versatility of application can develop to a broad spectrum of populations and problems.

REFERENCES

Evans, Ron L. & Jaurequy, Beth M. (1981). Group therapy by phone: A cognitive behavioral program for visually impaired elderly. *Social Work in Health Care*, *7* (2), 79-90.
Evans, Ron L. (1986). Cognitive telephone group therapy with physically disabled elderly persons. *Gerontologist, 26* (1), 8-11.
Evans, Ron L., Fox, Harold R., Pritzl, Denise O. & Halar, Eugen M. (1984). Group treatment of physically disabled adults by telephone. *Social Work in Health Care, 9* (3), 77-84.
Evans, Ron L. & Jaurequy, Beth M. (1982). Phone therapy outreach for blind elderly. *Gerontologist, 22* (1), 32-35.
Evans, Ron L., Kleinman, Leah, Halar, Eugen M. & Herzen, Kay. (1984). Predicting change in life satisfaction as a function of group counseling. *Psychological Reports, 55* (1), 199-204.
Evans, Ron L., Werkhoven, Walt & Fox, Harold R. (1982). Treatment of social isolation and loneliness in a sample of visually impaired elderly persons. *Psychological Reports, 51* (1), 103-108.
Jaurequy, Beth M. & Evans, Ron L. (1983). Short term group counseling of visually impaired people by telephone. *Journal of Visual Impairment and Blindness, 77* (4), 150-152.

Kennard, William W. Jr. & Shilman, Ruth Pollock. (1979). Group services with the homebound. *Social Work, 24* (4), 33-332.

Papell, Catherine & Rothman, Beulah. (1980, Summer). Relating the mainstream model of social work with groups to group psychotherapy and the structured group approach. *Social Work with Groups, 3* (2), 5-23.

Shilman, Ruth P. & Giladi, Beth H. (1985). Bridging the isolation gap: Making telephone connection. Special issue: Time as a factor in groupwork: Time limited group experiences. *Social Work with Groups, 8* (2), 134-137.